T0229730

"Only two years after the inception of the Covid-19 pandemic, Urmila Mohan produces a compelling account of the emotional, religious and subjective implications of this event. She investigates facial masks as micro-technologies of the self, revealing their imaginary dimension in sewing and making do geared to care, labor, religious practice, activism, loss, intimacy, boundaries. Bodies and materials in motion provide the rationale for a rich and striking iconography, expanding the scope of description and analysis of a crisis that is still unfolding."

Jean-Pierre Warnier, *Professor of Anthropology (retired), University Paris-Descartes, France*

"In this well written and exquisitely illustrated book on masks in motion, Urmila Mohan offers fascinating layers of insights into how people sew and use masks, and how the imperative to mask under the Covid-19 pandemic unmasked a myriad of vulnerabilities, tensions and cracks in the delicate and sensitive body of American society and politics."

Francis B. Nyamnjoh, *Professor of Social Anthropology, University of Cape Town, South Africa*

Masking in Pandemic U.S.

This anthropological study explores the beliefs and practices that emerged around masking in the U.S. during the COVID-19 pandemic. Americans responded to this illness as unique subjects navigating the flux of social and corporeal boundaries, supporting certain beliefs, and acting to shape them as compelling realities. Debates over health and safety mandates indicated that responses were fractured with varied subjectivities in play—people lived in different worlds and bodies were central in conflicts over breathing, masking, and social distancing. Contrasting approaches to practices marked the limits and possibilities of imaginaries, signaling differences and similarities between groups, and how actions could be passageways between people and possibilities. During a time of uncertainty and loss, the "efficacious intimacy" of bodies and materials embedded beliefs, values, and emotions of care in mask sewing and usage. By exploring these practices, the author reflects on how American subjects became relational selves and sustained response-able communities, helping people protect each other from mutating viruses as well as moving forward in a shifting terrain of intimacy and distance, connection, and containment.

Urmila Mohan is an anthropologist of material culture and religion with a focus on bodily practices. She is associated with the *Matière à Penser* group, is an Honorary Research Fellow in the Department of Anthropology, University College London, UK, and is the founder/editor of the open-access digital journal *The Jugaad Project*. She has researched and theorized materiality, praxis, and aesthetics in diverse contexts including religious communities and maker groups in India, Indonesia, and the U.S.

Routledge Focus on Anthropology

For more information about this series, please visit: https://www.routledge.com/anthropology/series/RFA

Masking in Pandemic U.S.

Beliefs and Practices of Containment and Connection

Urmila Mohan

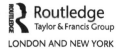

LONDON AND NEW YORK

First published 2023
by Routledge
4 Park Square, Milton Park, Abingdon, Oxon OX14 4RN

and by Routledge
605 Third Avenue, New York, NY 10158

Routledge is an imprint of the Taylor & Francis Group, an informa business

© 2023 Urmila Mohan

The right of Urmila Mohan to be identified as author of this work has been asserted in accordance with sections 77 and 78 of the Copyright, Designs and Patents Act 1988.

All rights reserved. No part of this book may be reprinted or reproduced or utilised in any form or by any electronic, mechanical, or other means, now known or hereafter invented, including photocopying and recording, or in any information storage or retrieval system, without permission in writing from the publishers.

Trademark notice: Product or corporate names may be trademarks or registered trademarks, and are used only for identification and explanation without intent to infringe.

British Library Cataloguing-in-Publication Data
A catalogue record for this book is available from the British Library

Library of Congress Cataloging-in-Publication Data
A catalog record has been requested for this book

ISBN: 9781032137629 (hbk)
ISBN: 9781032154251 (pbk)
ISBN: 9781003244103 (ebk)

DOI: 10.4324/9781003244103

Typeset in Times New Roman
by Deanta Global Publishing Services, Chennai, India

For those who cared for us during the pandemic.

Contents

Figures

Acknowledgments

As a study of practices, this project brings together people from diverse walks of life. My interlocuters are theater, film, costume, design, art and creative professionals. They are community activists, religious leaders and faith members, and educators and archivists. I am indebted to all for their generosity.

I am most grateful to Cheri Vasek, retired Associate Professor of Costume Design and Technology, University of Hawai'i, Manoa, and Monona Rossol, President/founder of Arts, Crafts and Theater Safety, Inc. for inspiring and advising me on core aspects of this book. I am also grateful to Kristina Wong, Performance Artist, Comedian and Elected Official, for sharing her insights on the organization and mobilization of the "Auntie Sewing Squad".

The following interlocuters have played a significant part in my research: David Arevalo, Clothier and costume designer; Ashley Bellet, Assistant Professor of Costume Design, Purdue University; Monica Bullard, Certified nurse-midwife and legal clerk/Member, Auntie Sewing Squad; Ronn Campbell, Senior Associate Professor of Theater, Columbia Basin College; Gianina Enríquez, Community Organizer, Queens Museum; Puneet Singh Gupta, Founder of Puneet Yoga/Member, Auntie Sewing Squad; Lily Hope, Alaskan Chilkat and Ravenstail weaver; Van Huynh, Member, Auntie Sewing Squad; Rev. Clare Johnson and Rev. Matthew Johnson, Fernwood Baptist Church; Vinnie Loucks, Costume technician and artist; Khammany Mathavongsy, Treasurer, Wat Lao Rattanaram, and community leader; Grace McEwan, Professional seamstress; Robin McGee, Costume designer, Broadway Relief Project; Norman Muñoz, Dancer and theater performer; Shannon O'Neill, Curator for Tamiment-Wagner Collections, New York University Special Collections; Lisa Perello, Seamstress and costume designer; Niceli Portugal, Family programs coordinator, Queens Museum; Giana Ricci, Librarian for the Fine Arts, Division of Libraries, New York University; Winnie van der Rijn,

Multi-disciplinary artist; Stephanie Cordova Rodriguez; Josephine (Jojo) Siu, Costume designer/Member, Auntie Sewing Squad; Jessica Smith, Prop artisan/Member, Broadway Relief Project; Ova Saopeng, Associate artistic director and producer, TeAda Productions/Member, Auntie Sewing Squad; Eliza West, Historical costumer; Jeff Whiting, President, Open Jar Studios, and Founder, Broadway Relief Project.

My appreciation to Shan Ayers and Trish Ayers, Laura Barclay, E. M. Chen, Madhavi Clark, Ryan Eller, Miranda Gast, Father Ilyas Gill, Peter Goldberg, Rosalind Guder, Christine Jeanjaquet, Deborah Nash, Frank New, Rae Robison, Valerie Snyder and Valerie Soe. A special note of thanks to Charles Grubbs and Margaret Grubbs, Fargofilms, and Dorian Coss, Director, for developing aspects of this research into the documentary "Common Thread". I remain indebted to neighbors, colleagues and friends who shared their reflections on the events of the past two years.

My sincere thanks to the Routledge editorial team. I am most grateful to those who commented on earlier drafts on this manuscript, including colleagues at a workshop held by "The Jugaad Project".

Introduction

Imaginaries, embodiment, and the U.S. covidscape

Introduction

Coronaviruses have become the foremost global public health threat of the 21st century. With the most reported confirmed infections of the novel coronavirus, COVID-19, the U.S. led the world in infection rates and deaths over 2020–2021.[1] Terms such as "next normal"[2] signaled a decisive shift in American society between a pre- and post-pandemic U.S. and the need for new resilient, imaginative practices to support the nation. Simultaneously, the virus's effects widened existing schisms of precarity and social inequity in a landscape where people moved cautiously to deal with the threat of sickness and loss (Figure 0.1). While the virus significantly changed culture, practice, and language around the world, this study focuses on the U.S. wherein cloth mask making was important in 2020 and 2021 due to the shortage of N95 masks or its equivalents. Stitchers mobilized to make tens of thousands of fabric masks and millions of people learned to incorporate masking into their everyday lives in a matter of weeks. The pandemic also led to peoples' heightened consciousness of embodied processes, such as breathing, and how bodies and materials helped them cope through sewing, worship, and various kinds of civic activities. This in turn led to the formation of, and engagement with, diverse analog and virtual community[3] spaces, ranging from physical sites for food banks to online networks for worship, mask making, and social activism.

This book focuses on how mask making and mask usage shaped Americans as subjects of the "covidscape." The concept of the scape is inspired by Appadurai's proposal of culture as the interaction of different kinds of scapes or imaginaries; where the world is "characterised by a new role for the imagination in social life" including "the French idea of the imaginary *(imaginaire)*, as a constructed landscape of collective aspirations" (1990: 4). Masking takes place in a pandemic world as it is being imagined,[4] and explicitly shaped by practices related to face covering. Practices are entangled with

DOI: 10.4324/9781003244103-1

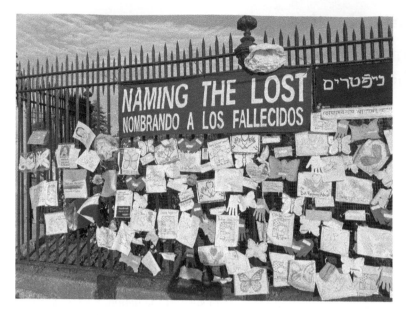

Figure 0.1 "Naming the Lost," a temporary installation that commemorates COVID-19 victims outside the Greenwood Cemetery. June 2020, Brooklyn, New York. Photo by author.

beliefs and affects, and the efficacy of ideas, images, and objects are worked through in the space of the imaginary to determine what is compellingly real or unreal. Part of this process is also contesting others' imaginaries. Shaped by a host of social factors, and embedded in affectively loaded perceptions and experiences, techniques of making and doing can be related to the flux of the imaginary where "it is always in the name of something *Real* that people are transformed into believers and are marched forward."[5] The real, in De Certeau's (1987) view, is not so from an ontological, universal, reified, point of view but is constructed as such by and for the believer. The persons who wear masks because they believe it is efficacious in preventing the virus and the persons who refuse to wear masks because they believe it cannot protect against the virus are appealing to different images ranging from what it is to be American to the usefulness of science. As Appadurai's (1986) influential volume on exchange and value proposed, things are person-like and their values emerge from social interactions between subjects and objects. That is, value emerges as a property of people and the politics that surround things-in-motion such that the ways people position themselves in order to gain, divert, or enclave value as power can be gleaned from practices.

Subjects, their objects, and their practices are important sites to explore how individuals, and activist and faith groups shaped, and were shaped by, face coverings as well as images of health, community, and creativity. Despite the common use of the term pivoting as a way to describe pandemic changes, Americans did not simply turn, adapt, and respond. In fact, the debates we saw over 2020–2022 were both an affirmation that responses were fractured with varied subjectivities in play, and that the body was central in all of these conflicts through breathing, masking, and social distancing. Certainly, masks evoked populist resistance in the U.S. both historically in the 1918 Spanish Flu[6] and today. But to focus simply on the debate between mask-compliers and deniers is to misunderstand the importance of dynamics of masking/unmasking where practices of imagination are social facts cohering communities (Durkheim 2008/1912). As the complex and varied responses to health protocols and mandates have indicated, Americans did not necessarily approach face coverings through their technical efficacy. Even those who supported masking had a rather shaky scientific understanding of masks' efficacy and relied on a range of interpretive and habitational practices (De Certeau 1984: xxii) to bridge this gap. The point to be made here is that all practices are entangled with beliefs, whether secular or religious, by virtue of an imaginary. Peoples' responses and notions of real are shaped by a host of social factors, embedded in affectively loaded perceptions and experiences. Moving away from the mask debate, what could we learn about the nature of belief from masks and the ways they connect with everyday practices as well as the formation of communities during the pandemic?

Based on interviews, digital and auto ethnography, and archival research, this book approaches masking and mask-making practices as subjunctive forces of motion, emotion, and transformation, where people practice both intimacy and distance, shifting between containment and connection as social, philosophical, and material forces, and the desire to make beliefs efficacious and compelling for oneself and others. While this study deals with the U.S., anthropological insights derived from analyzing imaginaries as fields of action and possibilities can be applied to understanding pandemic responses and their long-lasting effects, globally. The ideas developed in this book thus aim to add to the renewed consciousness of bodies' social role in the emergence of pandemic subjects and communities. Masking was a pandemic-induced practice that influenced and adapted relationships with social "pods" as well as numerous civic engagement projects, ranging from food distribution to health care to mask making that sought to create a sense of community. Quotidian social practices persisted during the pandemic through day-to-day and face-to-face, albeit masked, activities as people lived and moved between spaces. Issues of power and agency could be associated with masking and social distancing practices as they were very much embodied in the pandemic subject through skills, beliefs, and religio-politics. The pandemic subject is a habituated and habilitated entity who brings experiences and knowledge with them from other activities (quilting, acting, teaching, walking) but must also, during uncertainty, adapt this knowledge to relate desires for protection and progress (Figure 0.2).

A study of pandemic practices that pays close attention to how people sew and use masks can help us understand the relevance of containment and connection, intimacy, and distance as a means of living relationally, and incorporating concerns for self and other. The chapters in this book explore fluxes and flows of various kinds of making whether of practices, subjects, objects, or communities, and prioritize people's corporealized experiences and emotions to portray diverse Americans as feeling and acting subjects of the pandemic, negotiating between internal and external states, affects, and senses.

The people we meet in this book are of varied races, ethnicities, and diasporic origins as well as occupations, and are situated in different parts of the U.S. They include costume designers, civic engagement and activist

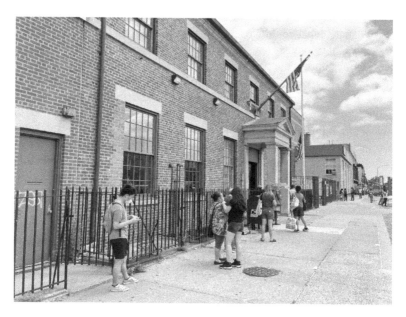

Figure 0.2 People maintaining social distance while waiting in line to enter a post office. July 2020, Brooklyn, New York. Photo by author.

groups, and faith groups, and we encounter them in spaces such as homes, businesses, stores, studios, temples, and churches. Many are caught in the paradox between American ideals of success through independence and hard work, and the ways in which social vulnerabilities and inequities have been exposed by the pandemic. Thus, the people we meet in this book draw upon multiple, intersecting imaginaries and a repertoire of existing practices and social relationships to deal with uncertainty, risk, and change. But how do they shift or adapt to navigate the pandemic? By studying subject–object interactions as entanglements of bodies, materials, and affects, this book looks at how practices (both secular and religious) shape images, values, and beliefs into something compelling, real, and actionable, similar to the way that religious praxis and rituals transform and propel the believer (Mohan and Warnier 2017).

Before proceeding further, it is worth noting that my experience as ethnographer was greatly influenced by experiences of closeness and distance in the pandemic. On one hand, social distancing and masking created a hunger for face-to-face social contact, putting bodies squarely back in the frame. On the other hand, people learned to rely on virtual media to satisfy their needs for interaction even as they chafed against the limits of technology. My research methodology was shaped by virtual media and social media in a sustained manner over 2020–2022, at least until the time the vaccine was widely available. My reliance on virtual means, such as Zoom, to interact with people around the U.S. echoed the global acceleration of video conferencing during the pandemic,[7] the plethora of new imaginaries that were facilitated, and the ways in which the virtual was incorporated or disincorporated with the analog. Indeed, one could say that the pandemic subjects studied through practices in this book are also digital subjects based on their affective and subjectivating relationships (Deleuze 1988 in Isin 2012: 77, Markham 2020) with devices, platforms, and digital forces. More accurately, these pandemic subjects are shifting inter-digital and trans-media subjects (Gershon 2010) as they move and relate across image and sound formats, and are shaped by technologies of communication such as video/audio chats, text messages, smart phone applications, and social media and networking sites. Observations and analyses of such media as practices and data sources will therefore be woven into some of the chapters in this book.

Practices as the making of subjects (and their objects)

As Appadurai's (ed. 1986) influential volume on exchange and value proposed, commodities are person-like and values of things emerge from social interactions between people and objects; that is, value emerges as a property of people and the politics that surround things-in-motion. In a context where the things being exchanged include both objects and people's desires for them (Appadurai 1986: 3), politics is the link between regimes of value and objects. The ways in which people position themselves and their objects in order to gain, divert, or enclave power can be gleaned from bodily practices whether centered in studies of material culture as subject-making or object-making.[8] This book focuses for the most part on subject-making and explores diverse groups through processes of imagining and believing[9] using dialectical relationships of motions and emotions.[10] It relies on a framework of ideas drawn from the anthropology of ritual and religion, globalization, embodiment, subjectivation, and material and visual culture. Motions of bodies, materials, and technologies have been covered previously through praxeological and phenomenological approaches in anthropology.[11] These streams are brought into dialog with the work of the *Matière à Penser* group on subjectivation as the incorporation of materials into bodies (Mohan and Douny eds. 2021; Mohan and Warnier 2017; Warnier 2007) and where a subject is always an entity in motion with its objects.

Practices are discussed as part of power and material flows that have effects on people and shape them as subjects. Such processes may also have unintended consequences through the types of diversions and tensions described above. From a Foucauldian perspective, subjectivation is an event that may or may not happen and is not determinate. Within this uncertain process, selves are the result of conscious and habitual process of identification (Bourdieu 1990) brought into dialog with felt selves (Damasio 2010: 185) and technologies of self (Foucault 1988). This notion of selves is incorporated into the pandemic subject via the body-in-motion. While the practice of masking may be inter-subjective due to actions of wearing the mask and perceiving another's mask, in order to consciously use the mask to create a community (Wenger 1998), the object must engage people in common activities. Materials are important as they have properties and aesthetic qualities that are sensed, perceived, and used as part of exchange flows of values within imaginaries. That is, the imaginaries explored in this book are mediated by images and practices and made compelling through praxeological and phenomenological incorporation in the practitioner's sensori-motor apparatus, feelings, and subjecthood.

Masks, distance, and intimacy

Most of the public discussion of masks' efficacy is centered around their technical ability to form permeable or impermeable barriers and to selectively allow entry and exit to breath, moisture, and virus-laden droplets. But masking is not just a protocol but a habit that is acquired over time through repetition of actions, perceptions, and responses with space for interruption, forgetting, and misplacing. The social efficacy of masks can vary from their technological efficacy, and the two can be aligned or misaligned through images and practices. That is, masks can be repurposed to fit with concerns that may or may not coincide with physical protection from the virus. By considering masks as a type of bodily paraphernalia or garment, we can better understand how they flexibly mediate various surfaces and contexts since they possess a dual quality. Masks act as mediating surfaces that touch the body but face outwards to society with their effects enmeshed in lived experience through inter-subjective values and practices.

Mask usage can be related to intimacies of various kinds as the ability to generate subjects through practices and beliefs. Apart from masks' ability to be technically efficacious and protect against the virus, states of distance or closeness are related to sustaining belief and relationships. For instance, this window of a Latinx art studio in Brooklyn (Figure 0.3) depicts a moment

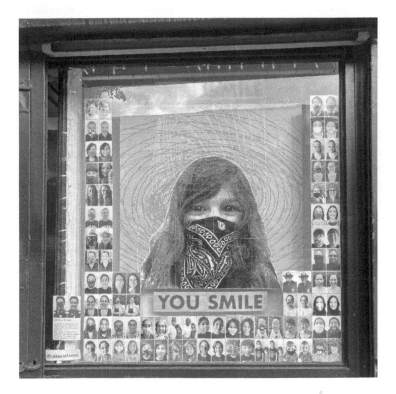

Figure 0.3 An art space window featuring photos of local residents. La Bodega Studios, Brooklyn, New York. May 2020. The studio was subsequently closed down. Photo by author.

in May 2020 when spaces were shut, social life was constrained, and people were feeling anxious and detached from each other. In a neighborhood that seemed ominously quiet, this window space displayed the faces of participants who were earlier asked to send in their pictures, both masked and unmasked. The resulting image in this case, both literally and metaphorically, was the invocation of a (hoped for) collective—a community of smiling faces eliciting feelings of solidarity and hope.

The question to be asked here is what objects such as masks *do* to people not only through agency (Gell 1998) of objects and images but also through subjects' transformative practices involving bodies and materials. This is not to say that masks possess an agency of their own, although several cultures certainly hold the view that objects can be enlivened, but that the (dis)incorporation of masks into subjects' corporeal schemas is best studied through practices, for instance, when people wear or sew cloth masks. Such practices are more akin to embodied, sensuous, and affective works in progress that use the generative capacity of habit for accommodation and coexistence (Wise and Velayutham 2014 in Nymanjoh 2017), while, conversely, the denial of relational public health practices relies on different habits of independence, self-containment, and autonomy. That is, masking is a way to explore unmasking in the U.S. to reveal how people relate to each other during crisis and what they value. To put it in practice-based terms, how are closeness and distance embodied in activities through dynamics of attaching and detaching, putting on and taking off, and holding and letting go as part of the "efficacious intimacy" (Mohan 2019, 2021) between selves and worlds?

By connecting masks, framed here as exemplary technologies of containment (Warnier 2006), with pandemic subject-making, I seek to challenge prevailing views of how face coverings work in inter-subjective practices. By going beyond masks as markers of paranoia, secretiveness, criminality, and/or undesirable ethnicity, the examples in this book indicate the cultural capacity of masks and making as mechanisms of creativity (Hallam and Ingold 2007), action, and belief, mobilizing social imaginaries, capacities, and capabilities. Even while recognizing that the medical face mask has its own distinct history (Lupton et al. 2021: 10–11) from, say, religious masks, there is a common thread since these are all face coverings in close proximity with the skin and body. The fabric masks studied in this book are placed in conversation with ideas on how bodily paraphernalia and cloth embody and wield affects and effects. Accordingly, the theoretical and analytical ideas I draw upon are related to the importance of studying cloth as objects of motion and emotion. In the context of devotional practices in Hinduism in India (Mohan 2019) and Indonesia (Mohan 2018), I had previously discussed cloth's role in creating affective and sensory experiences that transformed the bodies of dressmakers and weavers as well as the clothed. Unlike an identity label or tag that is attached to something after the fact, cloth and clothing is more productively approached as part of a relational practice that uses the corporeality of surfaces, whether on or off the body, to craft identity through connections and resemblances to other visual and material realms (Küchler and Were eds. 2005: xxii).

The transformative capability of bodies and materials in motion can be seen in various cultures. The liminal aspects of masks have been studied in Latin America, Africa, and Asia (Emigh 1996; Feder-Nadoff ed. 2022; Ross 2016; Shulman and Thiagarajan 1996; Turner 2017/1969) and when applied to Western contexts help us consider masked practices as transformative. Alfred Gell describes how in much of Polynesia and South America skin decorations are an integral part of persons, indissolubly linked to their humanity, sociality, and their mortal condition (1998: 194–195). He notes how social persona and subjectivity unite the two-dimensional character of graphic designs/tattoos imposed on the skin and the three-dimensional plastic form of the body. Such a logic could be extended from tattoos to any object in close proximity to the skin.

Masks' materiality both as containment of viral spread and a container of human form helps us understand how pandemic practices both distance and connect peoples. People experience feelings of containment, for example, when being limited to a space due to the virus, waiting at home for the vaccine shot, or constantly second-guessing their safety practices. Simultaneously, they manifest desires for connection through a range of activities, from postcard writing campaigns and protest gatherings to sewing or helping at food banks. Emotions are involved as "embodied thoughts" where the self is aware of being involved (Rosaldo 1984: 143), as well as pre-cognitive, bodily states where social and affective forces shape humans as subjects. Various studies on motions and emotions[12] enhance the study of COVID-19 masking practices to explore how Americans responded during pandemic[13] and the type of subjects that were formed. Further, there is a tension or play between the normative self (and its practices) that people aspire to and the way they are shaped by wider forces and institutions either consciously or unconsciously.

The people we meet in this book are encountered during a time of crisis and desire certain states and relationships in line with their values and beliefs. In Chapter 1, this book's premise of the importance of containment and connection is introduced through the analogy of breath, and by providing an overview of pandemics' embodied effects on subjects via daily practices and experiences. In Chapter 2, we meet lay mask makers who work both independently and collectively to design and sew fabric masks. Issues of social and technical efficacy as well as problems of responding to a mutating virus are factored into the gestures they use to make masks. In

Chapter 3, the frame is widened to include larger social mobilization efforts of mask makers and the ways they create community via images of justice and labor. Sewing is usually envisioned as craftwork but, in this case, is related to the making of politicized, gendered, and aestheticized imaginaries. In Chapter 4, the religious beliefs of a diasporic Lao-Buddhist group in California and a Baptist church in South Carolina are explored for the ways in which they relate contemporaneous events and concerns to precepts and rituals. Finally, the Conclusion moves the book's premise forward by asking what processes of masking and unmasking American subjects have revealed about the value of a politics of care.

Bodies and spaces are involved throughout as containers of emotions, beliefs, and actions in the making of pandemic selves and subjects. In this nexus, a desire for social connection is made as "a process of building and remaking relationships in order to achieve a balance between intimacy and distance" (Hay 2014: 31 in Nyamnjoh 2017). The notion of pandemic relationships being born out of containment and connectivity, intimacy, and distance entails daily work by individuals to enact concern for self and others. While this is a process that takes place even during non-pandemic times, there is a heightened attention to sociality and boundaries during a health and safety crisis. That is, uncertainty disturbs peoples' images of themselves and the world as well as their abilities to anticipate the world through their usual activities and routines. Beliefs and values take on a special significance in filling these gaps, guiding subjects through the uncertain, and embedding and shaping subjects within emergent worlds.

Notes

1 By 10 June 2020, confirmed cases in the U.S. passed 2 million and by 23 July 2020 that number had doubled. By 16 October 2020, that number had doubled again to 8 million. Subsequently, infections spiked to a peak in January 2021 and by 20 February 2021 passed 28 million. (Deaths were nearly at 500,000 in the U.S. by 20 February 2021.) In comparison, India and Brazil, the next in line, were at half or less than half that number for infections. See COVID-19 Dashboard at Johns Hopkins University, https://coronavirus.jhu.edu/map.html, last accessed 27 February 2021.
2 A term coined by the management consulting firm McKinsey & Company for the post-COVID-19 dramatic restructuring of the economic and social order in which business and society have traditionally operated. https://www.mckinsey.com/industries/healthcare-systems-and-services/our-insights/beyond-coronavirus-the-path-to-the-next-normal, last accessed 28 March 2022.
3 While past notions of community have been bound geographically, virtual community can be an "anchor, an already formulated notion of shared online space and communicative interaction" (Bowman-Grieve 2009: 990).

4 See Anderson (1991), Appadurai (1996).
5 De Certeau (1987, Chapter 1, Section 2, para.1) in Mohan and Warnier (2017: 374).
6 Historically, masks were protested during the 1918 Spanish Flu both in the U.S. (Witt 2020: 78-80) and abroad (Porras-Gallo and Davis eds. 2014: 206) as part of a multiplicity of narratives. In the American context, long-standing historical patterns reemerged in the early months of the pandemic with state and local divergence in coronavirus policies (Witt 2020: 112). The types of images and values attached to the virus, for instance, through memes, endorsed or ridiculed masks and other safety practices.
7 For example, Zoom's daily meeting participants grew from 10 million in December 2019 to 200 million in March 2020. https://blog.zoom.us/a-message -to-our-users, last accessed 27 February 2021.
8 See Gowlland (2017), Naji and Douny (2009), Wilkinson-Weber and Ory DeNicola eds. (2016).
9 See De Certeau (1984), Lovell ed. (1998), and Wenger (1998).
10 See Ahmed (2014), Berthoz (2000), Lindholm (2005), and Merleau-Ponty (2012/1945).
11 See Leroi-Gourhan (1993/1964), Lemonnier (1992), Marchand (2012), Mauss (2006/1935), and Merleau-Ponty (2012/1945).
12 See Barrett et al. (2007), Damasio (1999), Lutz (1986), and Lutz and White (1986).
13 For a brief comparison between the U.S. and India, see Mohan and Bora (2020).

References

Ahmed, S. (2014). *The Cultural Politics of Emotion.* Edinburgh: Edinburgh University Press.

Anderson, B. (1991). *Imagined Communities: Reflections on the Origin and Spread of Nationalism.* London: Verso.

Appadurai, A. (1986). "Introduction: Commodities and the Politics of Value." In A. Appadurai ed., *The Social Life of Things*, 3–63. Cambridge: Cambridge University Press.

Appadurai, A. (1990). "Disjuncture and Difference in the Global Cultural Economy." *Public Culture*, 2(1): 1–24.

Appadurai, A. (1996). *Modernity at Large: Cultural Dimensions of Globalization.* Minnesota: University of Minnesota Press.

Barrett, L. F., Mesquita, B., Ochsner, K. N. and Gross, J. J. (2007). "The Experience of Emotion." *Annual Review of Psychology*, 58: 373–403.

Berthoz, A. (2000). *The Brain's Sense of Movement.* Cambridge: Harvard University Press.

Bourdieu, P. (1990). *The Logic of Practice.* Stanford: Stanford University Press.

Bowman-Grieve, L. (2009). "Exploring 'Stormfront': A Virtual Community of the Radical Right, Studies in Conflict & Terrorism." *Studies in Conflict and Terrorism*, 32(11): 989–1007.

Damasio, A. (1999). *The Feeling of What Happens: Body and Emotion in the Making of Consciousness.* New York: Harcourt Brace.

Damasio, A. (2010). *Self Comes to Mind: Constructing the Conscious Brain*. New York: Random House.

De Certeau, M. (1984). *The Practice of Everyday Life*. Berkeley: University of California Press.

De Certeau, M. (1987). *Histoire et psychoanalyse entre science et fiction* [Kindle version]. Retrieved from Amazon.com.

Deleuze, G. (1988). *Foucault*. Minneapolis: University of Minnesota Press.

Durkheim, E. (2008/1912). *The Elementary Forms of Religious Life*. Oxford: Oxford University Press.

Emigh, J. (1996). *Masked Performance: The Play of Self and Other in Ritual and Theatre*. Philadelphia: University of Pennsylvania Press.

Feder-Nadoff, M. A. ed. (2022). *Performing Crafts in Mexico: Artisans, Aesthetics, and the Power of Translation*. New York and London: Lexington.

Foucault, M. (1988). "Technologies of the Self." In L. H. Martin ed., *Technologies of the Self: A Seminar with Michel Foucault*, 16–49. Amherst: University of Massachusetts Press.

Gell, A. (1998). *Art and Agency: An Anthropological Theory*. Oxford: Clarendon.

Gershon, I. (2010). "Media Ideologies: An Introduction." *Journal of Linguistic Anthropology*, 20(2): 283–293.

Gowlland, G. (2017). *Reinventing Craft in China: The Contemporary Politics of Yixing Zisha Ceramics*. Canon Pyon: Sean Kingston Publishing.

Hallam, E. and Ingold, T. (2007). "Creativity and Cultural Improvisation: An Introduction." In T. Ingold and E. Hallam eds., *Creativity and Cultural Improvisation*, 1–24. Oxford: Berg.

Hay, P. L. (2014). *Negotiating Conviviality: The Use of Information and Communication Technologies by Migrant Members of the Bay Community Church in Cape Town*. Bamenda: Langaa.

Isin, E. F. (2012). *Citizens Without Frontiers*. London: Bloomsbury.

Küchler, S. and Were, G. eds. (2005). *The Art of Clothing: A Pacific Experience*. London: UCL Press.

Lemonnier, P. (1992). *Elements for an Anthropology of Technology*. Ann Arbor: University of Michigan.

Leroi-Gourhan, A. (1993/1964). *Gesture and Speech*. Cambridge: MIT Press.

Lindholm, C. (2005). "An Anthropology of Emotion." In C. Casey and R. B. Edgerton eds., *A Companion to Psychological Anthropology: Modernity and Psychocultural Change*, 30–47. Malden: Blackwell Publishing.

Lovell, N. ed. (1998). *Locality and Belonging*. London: Routledge.

Lupton, D., Southerton, C., Clark, M. and Watson, A. (2021). *The Face Mask in COVID Times*. Berlin: De Gruyter.

Lutz, C. (1986). "Emotion, Thought, and Estrangement: Emotion as a Cultural Category." *Cultural Anthropology*, 1(3): 287–309.

Lutz, C. and White, G. M. (1986). "The Anthropology of Emotions." *Annual Review of Anthropology*, 15(1): 405–436.

Marchand, T. (2012). "Knowledge in Hand: Explorations of Brain, Hand and Tool." In R. Fardon, O. Harris, T. Marchand, C. Shore, V. Strang, R. Wilson and C. Nuttall eds., *SAGE Handbook of Social Anthropology*, 260–269. London: Sage.

Markham, T. (2020). *Digital Life*. Cambridge: Polity Press.

Mauss, M. (2006/1935). "Techniques of the Body." In N. Schlanger ed., *Techniques, Technology and Civilisation*, 77–95. New York: Berghahn Books.

Merleau-Ponty, M. (2012/1945). *Phenomenology of Perception*. London: Routledge.

Mohan, U. (2018). *Fabricating Power with Balinese Textiles*. Chicago: University of Chicago Press/Bard Graduate Center.

Mohan, U. (2019). *Clothing as Devotion in Contemporary Hinduism*. Leiden: Brill.

Mohan, U. and Douny, L. eds. (2021). *The Material Subject: Rethinking Bodies and Objects in Motion*. London: Routledge.

Mohan, U. and Bora, S. (2020). "'Mask Cultures' in the United States and India." *Anthropology News* website, 25 September 2020. https://doi.org/10.14506/AN .1506.

Mohan, U. and Warnier, J.-P. (2017). "Marching the Devotional Subject: The Bodily-and-Material Cultures of Religion." *Journal of Material Culture*, 22(4): 369–384.

Naji, M. and Douny, L. (2009). "Editorial." *Journal of Material Culture*, 14(4): 411–432.

Nyamnjoh, F. B. (2017). "Incompleteness: Frontier Africa and the Currency of Conviviality." *Journal of Asian and African Studies*, 52(3): 253–270.

Porras-Gallo, M. and Davis, R. eds. (2014). *The Spanish Influenza Pandemic of 1918–1919: Perspectives from the Iberian Peninsula and the Americas*. Rochester: Boydell & Brewer.

Rosaldo, M. Z. (1984). "Toward an Anthropology of Self and Feeling." In R. A. Sweder and R. A. LeVine eds., *Culture Theory: Essays on Mind, Self, and Emotion*, 137–157. Cambridge: Cambridge University Press.

Ross, L. M. (2016). *The Encoded Cirebon Mask: Materiality, Flow, and Meaning along Java's Islamic Northwest Coast*. Leiden: Brill.

Shulman, D. and Thiagarajan, D. (1996). *Masked Ritual and Performance in South India: Dance, Healing, and Possession*. Indiana: Indiana University Press.

Turner, V. (2017/1969). *The Ritual Process: Structure and Anti-structure*. New Brunswick and London: Aldine Transaction.

Warnier, J.-P. (2006). "Inside and Outside: Surfaces and Containers." In C. Tilley, W. Keane, S. Küchler, M. Rowlands, and P. Spyer eds., *Handbook of Material Culture*, 186–195. London: Sage.

Warnier, J.-P. (2007). *The Pot-King: The Body and Technologies of Power*. Leiden: Brill.

Wenger, E. (1998). *Communities of Practice: Learning, Meaning, and Identity*. Cambridge: Cambridge University Press.

Wilkinson-Weber, C. and Ory DeNicola, A. eds. (2016). *Critical Craft: Technology, Globalization, and Capitalism*. London: Bloomsbury.

Wise, A. and Velayutham, S. (2014). "Conviviality in Everyday Multiculturalism: Some Brief Comparisons between Singapore and Sydney." *European Journal of Cultural Studies*, 17(4): 406–430.

Witt, J. F. (2020). *American Contagions: Epidemics and the Law from Smallpox to COVID-19*. New Haven: Yale University Press.

1 Practices of containment and connection

Introduction

It was mid-October in 2020 when I decided to get tested for the Covid-19 virus. After many months of relative isolation, I had started venturing out into the neighborhood and there was the possibility I could be asymptomatic. The testing center was close by, within walking distance from my home in Brooklyn. As I waited in line, a wide range of people of different sexes, ages and ethnicities came by. A young man, dressed as a construction worker stopped at the entrance and anxiously asked the attendant if he could get a rapid test that day as his employer needed it the next day before he could start a new job. A young woman in navy blue scrubs, a medical worker perhaps, awaited her turn in the line with her head down, focused on her phone. After the test—a nasal swab which was not as painful as I had feared—I stopped at a bakery. A Hispanic family of four, father, mother, toddler son and baby in a stroller, paused outside the entrance. The little boy pulled out his disposable mask from his coat pocket with a practiced air and covered his nose and mouth with it as he entered the store. His father did the same. Then the mother pushed the stroller with the baby inside the bakery. The bakery owner reminded her to put on her mask and she complied while waiting at the door. There were signs in Spanish on the counters asking customers to clean their hands with sanitizer. The father walked across the room to use the dispenser before taking a tray and a pair of tongs to select baked goods.

The encounter described here took place in New York city well after it had reopened and when health protocols were widely known and generally practiced. The anecdote documents a moment when people in the city had become used to testing procedures and safety protocols in public spaces. The toddler knew the practice of entering a store involved putting on his

DOI: 10.4324/9781003244103-2

mask first. His mother entered without a mask, taking advantage of the open door to push the stroller inside, but quickly put hers on when reminded by the store owner. Her husband had read the signs and, even though he was using tongs, knew to use the hand sanitizer before approaching the baked goods. All of these activities, ranging from the ubiquity of getting COVID-19 tests to new sanitary practices, were ways of living in, and with, the pandemic.

People use practices to transition and cope with change, and learn to negotiate a world that they find confusing or scary. Such practices rely on bodies and spaces as material surfaces and "containers" both shaping, and shaped by, experience and perception (Warnier 2006, 2007: 54) and the "multisensoriality embedded in the materiality of human existence" (Howes 2006: 161). Phenomenologists have explored the subject as relating to the world through the body and the body as the being-in-the-world of the subject where the world is a field of awareness and meaning (Merleau-Ponty 2012/1945; Csordas ed. 1994, 1997). Here, practices manifest a way of interacting with, and feeling and experiencing the world through motion and emotion, as well as demarcating boundaries of sociality. Ways of being, feeling, and navigating spaces become part of imaginaries where the concept of an imaginary does not mean that people necessarily believe in something false or untrue. Rather, it indicates a space of indeterminacy or flux and "a *capacity* to produce images that will give their shape to tangible or intangible things and produce them as having some sort of compelling reality" (Salpeteur and Warnier 2013: 172, emphasis mine). This transformative potential of flux can be observed in how pandemic practices make new relationships by creating new boundaries and shifting old ones. To support this exploration of the covidscape as a generative realm of world-making,[1] the ideas of various scholars will be engaged including De Certeau's (1987) work on the historiographical uses of images in shaping people as believers of some kind, Appadurai's (1990, 1996) foregrounding of imagination in cultural scapes, and research on bodies, senses, and cognition.

Breathing as practice: Navigating pause and pivot

As part of his reflection on the mask as response and "response-ability," Wallace (2020: 340) evokes the palpable sense of uneasiness that was felt by Americans in the early days of the pandemic. Through observations of policy memos "that confuse respirators, masks, and pieces of cloth" and "mainstream media ... systematically refusing to provide its "sources"" even while citing science, he conjures the speed at which ambiguous and contradictory information shaped the rhetoric and anxiety surrounding masks. The slipperiness of imaginaries of health and safety reveals the tenuous hold that these had on reality. Paradoxically, uncertainty was heightened by information that was meant to clarify; for example, mask makers were unsure whether masks would be harmful and if they should make two-layered or three-layered masks, with or without filters.[2] Uneasiness suggests the importance of feelings as emotions and sensations, and the problem of making decisions in the face of uncertainty. Instead of relying on rationality, human risk calculation and decision-making regarding complex personal and societal problems rely on emotions whether encountered in internal or external worlds, images, or objects (Damasio 1994: 191; Douglas 1966;[3] Lupton 2013). Since precise calculation is impossible, especially when the phenomenon itself is changing, it is emotions such as fear, sadness, anger, and frustration, and the cultural ways in which they are expressed and perceived, that guide our decisions. That is, humans are feeling creatures who think and "emotion and feeling, along with the covert physiological machinery underlying them, assist us with the daunting task of predicting an uncertain future and planning our actions accordingly" (Damasio 1994: xiii). When combined with the *habitus* as the "schemes of perception, thought, and action" (Bourdieu 1977) that produce individual and collective practices, the body-in-motion as container of emotions, affects, desires, etc. can be related to events (infections, deaths, stages of the pandemic, mutations of the virus), and how they shape people as shifting subjects. Emotions can thus be related to the transformative power of "real, potent, and important aspects of conscious life and behavior" (Barrett et al. 2007: 390) as well as wider social affects and forces.

Pandemic events and effects lend themselves to the analogy of breath (Lupton et al. 2021) with stages of pause, or interruption of breathing, and pivot, or the resumption of breathing. Pause implies a distressing interruption of breath as motion, a hold on lives, and the reality of lost jobs and stalled routines. Many of my interlocuters referred to the early stages of pandemic as a pause, further articulated as a time of stasis and uncertainty. Unlike terms, such as lockdown, shutdown, and shelter-in-place, pause suggested an interlude and therefore a sense of anticipation of a post-pause period. As a corollary to pause, the term "pivot"[4] began to be used quite early in various contexts to the extent that it became a gloss for any (anticipated) resumption of activity. Businesses were lauded in the news for pivoting both literally and metaphorically. Artists used the term "bent knees"[5] to invoke their pre-existing ability to move and turn quickly much like in basketball or dance to come up with solutions to unanticipated problems. The notion of bent knees, ready to swivel and move in any direction, brings up the image of a body conditioned and prepared through a history of practice. Moving through the covidscape involved acquiring new skills and knowledge and using them to respond to pandemic uncertainty as, in one possible approach, the "disjuncture between territory, subjectivity and collective social movement" (Appadurai 1996: 188). Returning to the concept of response-ability, pivoting is not simply about agility but also includes peoples' access to resources, that is, in this analogy, the access to air as a medium that allows bodies to live and move. This is what Gibson called an "affordance" (1979: 15) as a way to unite the possibilities or opportunities in nature, and how people perceived and enacted them. Extending this to pandemic social events, Americans responded to the presence or absence of air, and changes and gaps induced by the pandemic in the religious, political, or economic realm as specific kinds of subjects.

The virus drew our attention to the fraught activity of breath, and how respiration and filtration are critical activities as we monitor contagion and transmission of disease. In breathing as a life-sustaining and affective practice, changed rhythms of respiration accompany our slide into slumber and, conversely, arousal into awakened states of desire and action. Breathing also takes place in conjunction with materials. Wearing a mask over our noses and mouths is a barrier as well as tactile stimulation, making us conscious of our breath—its smell, its warmth, and its moistness. Breath becomes a haptic tool of sociality and spirituality (Kearney 2021), a way to get in touch with ourselves and others. Breathing is a means of connection as well as a way to identify sensory and social boundaries between persons and groups. We are physically and emotionally close with those whose breath we share, that is, we literally breathe the same air, and distanced from people whom we consider as different and not part of our race, class, or cultural sensorium (Le Breton 2017: 97, 164). This sense of distance was vividly conveyed in dramatic events such as the Black Lives Matter (BLM) protests (Figure 1.1) wherein images of breathing were channeled through the slogan "I can't breathe"—first uttered by numerous Black people, most recently by George Floyd, before they died in law-enforcement encounters. These events illustrated that diverse and sometimes conflicting imaginaries of justice, nationhood, and American citizenship relied not only on ideology but a sensorial, affective and material framework that united some people while dividing others into ideal/non-ideal subjects. Drawing on Anderson's (1991) notion of the imagined nation, Morgan (2007: 165) notes how 19th to 20th century visual imagery in the U.S. relied on the power to evoke "symbolic sensations in the minds and bodies of its citizens." Most people never met physically but were entangled through these mediatized forms in debates over American identity and beliefs.

The re-imagining of the American as subject and nation continues today, relying both on the power of actual bodies and materials, and on the ability to abstract and represent these tangible entities (and associated meanings) through images. Underlying this is the politics of breath as symbols and

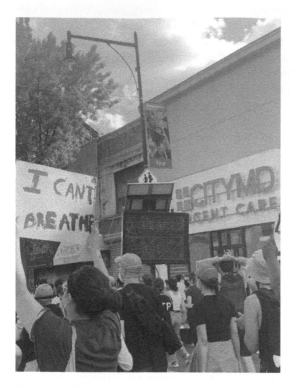

Figure 1.1 BLM protests in New York. The electronic sign by the city urges people to wear masks while protestors hold signs with the slogan "I Can't Breathe." June–July 2020. Photo courtesy of Sophia Gallagher.

practices that facilitates or constrains certain ways of living and being over others. The image of a free and self-determining citizen has been (re)presented and pursued as an ideal in the U.S., despite the "American Paradox" (Du Bois 1915: 709) of a nation that has been dematerialized since its inception in starkly inequitable ways. The existence of some bodies is clearly valued over that of others, for instance, through race, gender, and immigration preferences. Therefore, it is unsurprising that the most vocal anti-masking sentiments align with a demographic that is white, conservative, and nationalist, and used to possessing "privileges of subjectivation" (Bertrand 2021; Perry et al. 2020) in the U.S.

Freedom of thought and choice prevail in Americans' decision-making whether it is food habits (Rozin et al. 2011) or health protocols (Timpka and Nyce 2021). These preferences indicate not only how Americans diverge in their attitudes and beliefs from, say, Europeans, but also signal what type of symbolic and practical elements of experience carry weight in pandemic experience. A pragmatist attitude where ideas are judged based on practical outcomes means that Americans expect science to be instrumental, giving them real-world solutions that are practicable, immediate, and unambiguous. A public health discourse that does not meet these assumptions may fade into the background in favor of narratives that stabilize the virus, for instance as a single COVID-19 virus that does not mutate or change. Against this backdrop, health practices such as wearing a mask or being inoculated with a newly developed vaccine becomes one more instance of exercising pragmatism. When associated with ideological viewpoints and the role of emotions, such as the foundational myths of the U.S. based on a Protestant work ethic and anger over state mandates, mask contestation becomes a way to assert individualism and/or independence from the government while blaming those who do fall ill for a lack of control, bad habits, racial pre-dispositions, etc. The virus thus creates ruptures and exposes gaps in peoples' perceptions in the covidscape wherein there is a moral and emotional judgment attached to health and practices (Whorton 1982), and the pandemic becomes an event because this is when Americans recognize that imaginaries of safety, belonging, and equity are in conflict within the nation.

Shaping the self through an awareness of breath

The feeling and thinking body stores information from past experiences as behaviors even as it is "constantly being molded by the practices it executes" (Scheer 2012: 201). Face coverings as well as the experiences of mask makers can be approached as materially engaged activities that generate and create change through transformative experiences.[6] Throughout this book, practices are approached as ways of transforming subjects as well objects, that is, ways of doing and making things that transform mask stitchers/mask users as well as face coverings.

In an early Zoom chat in August 2020, I conversed with Michael,[7] a Chicano costume technician and graduate student who lived in Chicago with his husband, and Sarah,[8] a white theatrical costumer from North Carolina who shared a residence with her husband. Both were in their 30s and people I had identified as mask makers, also sharing a common social media network. The discussion was a way for Michael and Sarah to introduce themselves to each other beyond their interactions on Facebook, and they quickly established further commonalities as people who "came from the South." Both expressed the sentiment that they were used to (and exhibited) an attitude of friendliness, presented as a cultural trait of Southerners. I asked Michael and Sarah to assess the applicability of the term pause to their experience and while both had heard the term, Sarah said that it was "too clean" whereas her experience was one of limbo. She was in "full hum of active work" preparing for a show that was to open and then there was a sudden drop and "loss of direction." At first, she was unsure, confused about the views she found on social media about the efficacy of masks. Making masks for her family after two weeks of quarantine restored a sense of normalcy to her day that had been missing. When she realized that her rent was due and her unemployment check had not yet come, it forced her to revive her Etsy store and become an entrepreneur. What followed wasn't just one pivotal moment but multiple moments or shifts wherein Sarah had to make new decisions about both her store and her responses to unfolding political events.

Michael described pivot as a time that made him "paranoid" and "anxious" to leave the house. He spoke of how he made a set of masks in March as an initial response to the shutdown. Like Sarah he was unsure if the masks he made would help or hurt, describing it as the pressure of "Am I doing the right thing?" He made enough so that he could sleep knowing that his family had two masks a piece. As a first-generation college student, Michael came from a lower income, Chicano community in Texas, and the highest level of education in his family was high school. Part of the "panic" he dealt with was finding out that his parents were sharing a mask or reusing them, and having to emphasize how masks were to be used. In these comments, Michael's feelings were explicit. The terms he used (pressure, panic) were affectively charged and his emotions were visible in his bodily gestures. While we talked Michael moved his hands constantly, playing with synthetic slime and constantly moving it from one hand to the other. There were multiple pivotal moments in Michael's statement or what we could think of as markers by which he remembered and relived his mask-making and mask-wearing experiences. He discussed a significant moment where he made a limited edition of masks as political statements or "message masks." His 45 "message masks" made in June and July 2020 had Black Lives Matter (BLM) messages printed on them in text and dialogued with issues of race and identity in the U.S. Michael's language continued to be emotionally charged when he spoke of his "rage and helplessness" about anti-maskers who were chanting "I can't breathe" as a rebuttal to mask mandates. "And the idea that you would co-opt the death of a black man to help fill your mission was unimaginable to me. I felt I had to do something about that part!"

As we came to the end of a long conversation, Michael shared that although he hated the experience of wearing masks due to the way it hid facial expressions, "it was survivable" and he wore the ones he made as a "political act" of empowerment. In fact, the only masks he wore were the message masks but he first had to undergo an act of "conversion" and self-conviction to be comfortable with displaying his politics on his face. By comparison, Sarah remained reticent to share her views on social media. Coming from a conservative Christian culture, she described it as the dilemma of being a young woman in the arts but also living in the "deep" South where she "hid" some of her "crazy" family members on her Facebook timeline.

> The stakes just keep going up. For several years this whole divide has been going on in our country and its been getting further and further apart. ... But I'm not gonna change them so am I supposed to fight with my family every time we have dinner? No, I don't want to! ... For me, all I can do is wear my mask.

At one tense moment, Sarah was silent for about three to four seconds as she shed tears about this conflict. In a subsequent conversation, she acknowledged that Michael was "not wrong" in asking her to be more open about her politics but she remained hesitant. Nearly, six months later when perusing her Facebook feed, I noticed that something had changed. A day after the Capitol insurrection on 6 January 2021, she had posted a heartfelt message condemning white supremacy disclosing her feelings of "disgust and broken heartedness" at the "hatred and ignorance" in the U.S. Several "likes" on this post indicated that at least some members of her virtual social circle supported her views.

To return to an earlier moment in August, Michael and Sarah had overlapping interests from being in the theater world. But their situation and the varying intersectionality of their politics had influenced the way they pivoted. Their difference in views on masks' purpose and whether it should be implicit or explicit opened into a larger narrative over the American political landscape. But this was not simply one of being pro- or anti-masking. On one level both Michael and Sarah said that all they could do was "wear a mask" and that it was a deeply personal decision. Yet, the level of social risk they were willing to take in associating other types of images with masking varied depending on the type of imaginary they were embedded within. In Michael's case an activation of the mask as pro-BLM solidarity was possible due to his own previous marginalization as a queer Chicano man but a process of self "conversion" was also required. In Sarah's case since family peace took priority, political beliefs did not translate into an explicit stand until much later.[9]

Practices are skillful behaviors that are either learned or have become automatic. The people I spoke with over the pandemic were navigating their own uncertain worlds where closeness and distance, masking and unmasking, and the ability to pivot and adapt acquired new significance even while continuing to fold in older attitudes and habits. Some practices were more expressive, for instance, in the way Michael handled synthetic slime to control his anxieties and Sarah shed quiet tears over the conflict in her family. Both of these instances could be considered visible forms of "emotion work" or the way in which we "hold" feeling—how loose, how tight, how reluctant, how keen" (Kemper 1990: 122) evidenced during the highly relational and social act of conversing. In other instances, this holding (and release) of feeling could be related to Michael's deliberation on when he was ready to literally wear his politics on his face and, in Sarah's case, the conscious act of displaying a Facebook post on her timeline to mark a change in self and affiliation. The events of the pandemic were experienced and narrated differently, including the ways they related to the BLM protests. While this was a cause close to Michael's heart, Sarah remained silent on this issue, preferring to situate her masks as "just" a physical need. Since Sarah's willingness to declare her beliefs on social media took place later, it is worth noting that the types of responses elicited were constantly shifting and indicative of a pandemic flux of changing events, narratives, and images. To use the analogy of breathing as a way to contain and connect, Sarah's and Michael's views were also part of an imaginary, bridging unique biographical concerns as well as wider affective forces such as the BLM protests and the Capitol insurrection.

Creating and navigating boundaries

Breath and its organs, such as the nose and throat, are liminal spaces between internal and external realms where substances in the body begin to come into contact with what is ingested. This may also be why breathing and associated actions, such as swallowing food or chanting on prayer beads, are considered ritualistic practices in many cultures (Mohan 2016; Nyamnjoh and Rowlands 2013) and techniques of monitoring physical and spiritual boundaries. When considering how people move through the covidscape, we encounter a body of practices, including but certainly not limited to the preparation to leave home and enter public spaces, hand washing, maintaining social distance, paying attention to government-mandated rules, washing masks after use, etc. Could the analogy of breathing as a way to understand flux and transformation be applied to these practices as well? The stories below are of some different survivors whose recovery was entangled with the development of new boundaries and how to maneuver them through actions of ingestion and egestion, and containment and connection. Containers of various kinds and sizes were involved in the process, ranging from the human body and its paraphernalia to rooms, homes, restaurants, and neighborhoods.

The first account is located in a Mexican-American restaurant in Brooklyn that I frequented during my walks, first for hydrating juices over summer, and later for outdoor dining over fall and winter 2020. It was the day after Thanksgiving in the end of November 2020, and with a combination of Mexican pop and Christmas music playing in the background, I chatted with Maria and her mother Rosa in their restaurant. Since her mother only spoke Spanish, Maria translated on her behalf. The father ran a bodega or convenience store next door and I had heard stories from Maria over the summer of how he had been physically threatened by a customer for enforcing masking rules. We had maintained a line of communication until this time when we had a long conversation about their pandemic experiences.

Rosa was in her 40s and had four children, including her eldest daughter Maria who was in her early 20s. Maria, along with her siblings, helped with the restaurant and translated as well as implemented the changing government rules around COVID-19 dining. Under the protective gaze of a figure of St. Jude, a table was covered with thick binders containing records of employee health screens, cleaning and disinfecting logs, and contact tracing forms from diners, as well as an infrared thermometer, hand sanitizer, and wipes. This section also acted as a barrier between customers and the cashier. Similar concerns with boundaries, and what was a safe distance, were being enacted in the outdoor seating area. New York city's restrictions on dining, schools, businesses, and houses of worship followed a color coding by "cluster zones,"[10] which were intended to help control COVID-19 spread and protect hospital capacity. Accordingly, dining regulations kept changing with the fluctuating infection rate over 2020 and 2021, and rules were constantly being updated; information sometimes came in mere hours before new rules were implemented.

The definition of what constituted outdoor seating was vague and costly to implement, and at the time of this conversation, in late November 2020, the family had placed several tables outside the restaurant within a roofed structure with plexiglass walls on three sides. (A later rule mandated that a raised floor had to be created for this structure if it was to be safe in winter.) When I followed up with them in early December 2020, this structure was regarded as indoor seating in the new rules, and Maria had received the notice that they would have to reduce the number of tables outside if they were to continue using the space. Along with this confusion over outdoor/indoor as categories of activity, the family was facing problems of being in public-facing roles where they had to translate and mediate between unwilling customers and government mandates. For instance, when this area in Brooklyn was coded yellow in December 2020, there was resistance from customers demanding to be seated at the same table with the rest of their group whereas the rules only permitted four people at one table. According to Maria, people would get upset and try to resist the rule by joining tables so that they could be seated together.

Maria's parents had emigrated to the U.S. from neighboring villages in Puebla state in Mexico. Only her mother's father was left there and, at the time of the interview, her father's parents were still alive in the U.S. (Both grandparents unfortunately succumbed to COVID-19 about three months later.) Rosa spoke of getting sick twice, first in March and then in April 2020. Her husband and children also fell ill. Maria was fortunate as she had mild symptoms and got better fast. Rosa had constant fever in the beginning along with coughing and body ache that would not let her sleep anywhere except upright in a chair. The family restaurant was closed and didn't reopen till the beginning of May. While she was ill and after she recovered, Rosa remained worried and anxious about how she would take care of her family and the business.

In the context of suffering and death that Rosa had witnessed in the Mexican and Latinx community, it seemed that her source of strength was her faith in the Virgin of Guadalupe, whose figure was situated in a high alcove in a corner of the restaurant (Figure 1.2) furthest away from diners

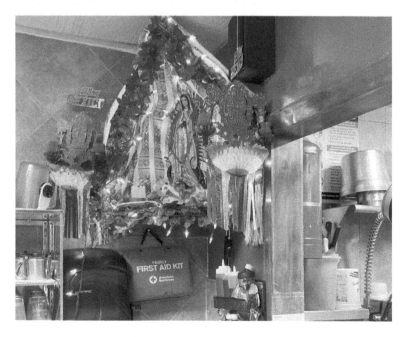

Figure 1.2 An altar in Rosa's restaurant is dressed up to celebrate the Virgin of Guadalupe's birthday. A kitchen can be seen to the right. Brooklyn, New York. December 2020. Photo by author.

and easily accessible to family members. This effigy had been brought over from the Basilica of Our Lady of Guadalupe in Mexico City, and was clothed and taken care of by Rosa regularly. It wore a rosary that had been given by the church to the family when they "received" the Virgin in the restaurant. Rosa was the main family member who took care of the altars also setting up the Day of the Dead altar *(ofrenda)* in the restaurant that year for her own mother. She showed me a photo on her phone, explaining the various offerings and the sequence of events as well as the days when the souls of the departed arrived and left. One of the rituals was to leave a white candle at the door so that the soul would know which way to leave the house; marking the importance of liminality and borders in a way that refracted the family's current concerns with indoor and outdoor regulations.

Rosa's faith in the saints was strong and her belief in the Virgin pre-dated COVID-19 as somebody who, as Maria translated, "always delivered." Rosa had health problems before COVID-19 and was told there might be a cancerous tumor in her head. Going past the church one day for a medical test she asked the Virgin for help. The results later showed that she was fine and Rosa promised the Virgin she would be at church on 12 December 2019, to help celebrate the Virgin's birthday; in 2020, however, she would not be attending church on this day due to the dangers of COVID-19. Priests had started re-administering mass in churches but there was also the very real problem of where bodies were to be buried. It was rare to find people in the community with the resources to get buried in Brooklyn and so people went to a cemetery in the neighboring state of New Jersey because it was the only place they could afford. In this sense, everything about peoples' lives had been drastically changed by the virus and Maria described it as a process of taking it one day at a time. As a thoughtful, sensitive young woman, she spoke of how numerous people they knew had passed away and that she wasn't ready to attend mass memorials or funerals. Over multiple conversations and text message chats with her spanning many months, I sensed that while she maintained a calm front, the succession of deaths in her family, including the loss of her grandparents, had left their mark. Unlike her mother, however, Maria found solace by turning to political activism and participation, campaigning for a Latinx mayoral candidate, and finding employment with a Latinx candidate for New York Council District. She had also changed her educational plans from a Masters in music business to law, in the hope of helping her community. While acknowledging the loss of her grandparents on Instagram with a beautiful photo of the elderly couple, she mostly posted videos and photos of herself as a single, happy, care-free, young woman. In many of these images, the restroom in the restaurant became a private, performance space to go maskless and pose while sharing a new outfit, makeup style, or haircut. In this way, Maria was able to sustain a space of her own even while at work and shaped a virtual narrative of buoyancy and optimism.

The issues that Maria and Rosa faced in dealing with shared spaces and how to categorize them remind us that the problem of *how* to navigate an area is a concern even in domestic spaces, especially for those living in multi-storeyed buildings. Changing practices affected me as well as my neighbors in an apartment building in Brooklyn where different generations lived together. Many residents in this building were born and raised here. The population was slowly aging with the elderly moving to nursing homes, and their adult children moving away and selling their apartments to new inhabitants. Before the pandemic, it was common to see elderly women gathered outside the building for their regular evening chats. The virus, however, changed the way we socialized outside and inside the building, and every new rule or piece of information about the virus penetrated our lives in the form of signs, regulations, and increased vigilance about personal and shared spaces. Building management had made masks mandatory and tensions occasionally erupted into grievances, for example, over children making noise in the courtyard. Decisions were constantly being made about whether to enter an elevator with somebody else, or pause while somebody collected their mail and moved on, for fear that passing them would risk closeness. Risk calculation was very much an individual or family affair as the pandemic waxed and waned. For some, outdoor activity was limited to necessary trips to grocery stores (Figure 1.3), doctors, and for exercise, while others returned to gyms and indoor dining or gathered with family members during holiday celebrations.

Conversations about COVID-19 practices with my neighbors Isabel and Saul started as encounters in the building. Meeting Saul in the elevator one day, an exchange of pleasantries led to a discovery of his utter boredom and his enthusiasm to talk. He volunteered that he had fallen ill with COVID-19, donated plasma a few times, and would be happy to share his experience of, and recovery from the virus. Isabel lived across from me with her husband and two children and our conversation was prompted by a grocery delivery in early 2021. The boxes of produce and dried goods were left outside her door and she stood at the entrance with Lysol wipes in hand, wiping down each package before it entered the apartment. We chatted about her experiences that weekend over a coffee at a time when she could get away from her work and family responsibilities. Prior to my coffee chat with Isabel (held outside the café for safety reasons), I had built a narrative of events over 2020, noting her attention to disinfecting the door handles and elevator buttons every evening in March 2020 to the weeks over summer when it seemed that her entire family was in quarantine. As neighbors, it was clear

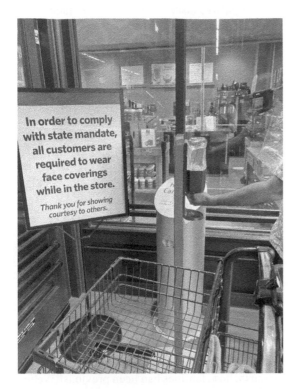

Figure 1.3 Shopping during the pandemic involved new practices of using hand
sanitizer and wiping down cart handles. Brooklyn, New York. July 2020.
Photo by author.

that there were times when she had food delivered and her mail collected
by another neighbor. Thus, seeing her wipe down groceries in January 2021
was an opportunity to both revisit these events and find out which practices
had persisted or changed.

It turned out that food was now a central issue for Isabel as she had
become a COVID-19 "long hauler," developing allergies in addition to
numerous other ailments, such as psoriasis and lack of energy. In her 40s
and normally active and energetic, Isabel had caught the virus early in the
pandemic, and had subsequently seen a cardiologist, neurologist, pulmo-
nologist, and, now, was consulting a nutritionist. Over the last year she had
suffered from shortness of breath, brain fog and forgetfulness, and anxiety
and depression. The psoriasis on her scalp had become a problem to the
extent that she cut her hair extremely short for relief. New habits had taken
over and Isabel jokingly referred to them during the conversation at various

times as a form of obsessive-compulsive disorder and post-traumatic stress disorder. Neither terms were intended as diagnostic but were instead meant to signal her high level of stress, her fear of exposure to the virus, and the way her life had been disrupted.

> Things have changed me completely. I can't put items into the freezer without cleaning them. I have my steps and there are things I have to do. If I go out and there are a lot of people around, I get home and take off my clothes, take a shower, and wash my hair whether it makes sense or not. When my kids come home from school they know the drill—go to the shower. They may think I'm crazy but they do it.

In another instance, Isabel narrated how she drove into the parking lot of a grocery store, panicked, and left because it was two in the afternoon, and she felt there were too many people in the store. She described these as a combination of things that she has always been vigilant about but also as issues that she had previously never paid attention to. For instance, "if I see people walking too close to each other, I immediately tense up." Unlike earlier, she could no longer simply take on a chore without advance calculation. Trips to the store had to be planned for early morning and times when the store would be less busy. Similarly, if the family went outdoors it would be to the park or to an open-air space. Her husband worked from home and her children (who were at the time attending school) were only allowed to socialize with a few companions whose families had been previously vetted for their safety habits.

What frustrated Isabel, like a lot of other people I spoke to, was not knowing where she caught the virus. She was constantly retracing her motions and those of her family, all of whom caught the virus except for her husband. Isabel reported getting ill two times, once in March 2020 for about a week and once in May for 27 days which, relying on her knowledge of software from her day job, she documented in an Excel spreadsheet. She described this as a time when she was confined to her room with nothing to do. "I lost my sense of taste and smell and the sense of time. My spreadsheet was what kept me going." With little to alleviate her pain and suffering apart from Tylenol, Isabel did her own research on how to feel better, identifying exercises for the back and lungs that she found on YouTube, getting advice from friends in Spain about the right duration for quarantine (40 days instead of 14, following the original meaning of the term), and using herbal tips from her mother in Puerto Rico. Even through the worst of her illness, Isabel continued to worry about her family. For example, every time she used the bathroom she would clean it down so as not to infect the others. After we returned from our coffee, this attitude of worry and her struggle with maintaining family responsibilities became more evident. As I had been temporarily locked out of my apartment, Isabel allowed me to enter her house and directed me to her kitchen where we continued to wear our masks as we chatted for 10–15 minutes. Having made sure that her 13-year-old son was attending his virtual piano classes and that her 11-year-old daughter was fed breakfast, Isabel returned to continue her conversation with me. Pointing to a half empty carton of cereal on the counter, she emphasized that things had changed and that the rest of the family was responsible for buying their own groceries. There was a list on the fridge where they could jot down what they needed but as of yet, she noted with exasperation, nothing had been entered. She was also trying to get her teenage son to do more chores around the house. What was underlined repeatedly in different ways during my time with Isabel was that things could not go on the way they had before as she had to concentrate on her own needs. At the time of writing, she was struggling with the process of re-learning how to eat due to food allergies and this took all of her energy and focus. She had eliminated dairy and gluten and was feeling stronger and healthier. She continued to cook for her family with a sense of smell that "comes and goes," relying on her recipes and habits.

The second vignette is drawn from my conversation with Saul who, like Isabel, lived on the same floor as me. Whenever I had spoken with him in the past, he had been quite willing to share his views on things, positioning himself as both knowledgeable and opinionated. Before the pandemic, I would generally meet Saul on his way back from work, still wearing his tour guide jacket from his job as part of a New York tour company. My conversation with him took place in his apartment in November 2020 when vaccines were not available. We sat in a room crowded with furniture and a large television panel with a graphic of swimming fish. After his two elderly cats had investigated me, he sat in his new La-Z-Boy recliner while I perched some distance away on the couch. Like Isabel, Saul reported having fallen ill twice but unlike her, he was less concerned about being re-infected by the virus. In his early 60s, Saul had been a tour guide in Manhattan for decades, had caught the virus in April 2020, and was now furloughed from his company. The tourism, hospitality, convention service, and live entertainment industries were shut down and he was suffering from the lack of fellowship and community. He was also "scared and depressed" that the tourism industry might never recover. Like Isabel, Saul had tried to retrace his steps to find out where and when he had been infected; it could have been while riding the subway, working on buses with travelers from throughout the world, or shopping in crowded stores before the mask mandates and social distancing. Since his aged father had passed away around the time when he fell ill, his COVID-19 story was entangled with that of his father's. He was frightened that he might have given the virus to his father and a good part of our conversation involved Saul reviewing dates and events on his phone and reasoning (more to himself than me) how with "twenty–twenty hindsight" he could not have transmitted the virus to his father. To explain the effects of the virus on his own body, Saul shared his step counter on his smart phone that illustrated how his last long walk was on 4 April 2020. After that he "crashed" and could not get a deep breath. Unable to move around the apartment, he was prone to violent, coughing fits and burning sensations when he took a breath. Like Isabel he had a second episode in mid-July where he fell ill and was unable to recover his earlier stamina or lung capacity for a long time. He described how his joints were inflamed and every shoulder muscle was "locked," and how he was feeling the effects of falls from years ago.

Saul's verbal responses to the virus were as complex as its physical effects. He was fearful of "self-doubt and imagining things, reading and imagining" but also referenced numerous New York Post articles[11] and con- spiracy theories that the virus was man-made in a Chinese lab and that it wasn't possible to have decades of research for developing a vaccine if it was supposed to be "brand-new." This comment, made at a time when vaccines were under media scrutiny, echoed a story that had been circulat- ing in the media since the start of the pandemic and had been repeatedly debunked.[12] Saul believed he had caught the virus in a public space where nobody was masking and with the high probability that it was transmitted during physical interactions with tourists from Europe. Yet, it was peoples' "personal responsibility to protect our individual exposures" and he was "bothered" that he *had* to wear a mask especially since he now considered himself to be immune to the virus. His claim that he didn't need to mask relied on a type of knowledge gap, bridged by the belief that his antibody level would remain high and he would not or could not be re-infected by the virus. When this assurance articulated with emotions, such as fears of permanent economic downturn and depression over the lack of community, it helped reinforce a way of living and responding to the uncertainty of a pandemic world. Saul described (and enacted) the debilitating side effects of the virus as he experienced them showing how his body would bend and contort during a coughing fit. While he maintained that nothing had changed about him "as a person," on further questioning he shared that "everything feels different on the inside. If I'm sweating, it smells different from before. … I lost my appetite and I'm sensitive to things and feel them different." Hesitantly narrating the effects of the virus, Saul was questioning what he knew about himself and the world, and our conversation captured a moment when he was trying to determine if the virus was just "another" health con- cern. Saul's comments indicated a type of flux that was intimately felt and mediated by the body, and a process by which he was trying to determine what was real and unreal when it came to the origins of the virus, whether to mask, and to what extent the government could mandate such practices. Such views were certainly not isolated and existed as part of a spectrum. For example, in casual conversations with neighbors who lived just a few floors from each other, I would hear comments laden with emotions, ranging from anxiety to calm, depending on whether the virus was perceived as a serious threat decimating people or "just" a kind of flu.

Apart from the disruption to lives caused by the virus, what is common in these diverse COVID-19 experiences is the centrality of the body and the manner in which various senses and emotions are invoked in narrating experience.[13] That is, how the existence of the virus penetrates peoples' lives as well as bodies; a potentially transgressive act that challenges subjectivity and society. Managing boundaries between subject and object, and between human and virus becomes a daily pre-occupation whether manifested in politicians using the language of war to speak of responses to the virus or interlocutors who noted that "everything feels different on the inside." Simultaneously, boundaries were being heightened, diverted, and challenged through daily practices indicating their varying beliefs and values.

Thinking about people as sensing and feeling entities allows us to relate subjects and objects to their material and visual culture and the ways they inhabit and cross spaces. When it comes to the experiences of Isabel, Saul, Maria, and Rosa,[14] varied spatial boundaries are present and can be accommodated under the paradigm of embodied practices and experiences. This includes biographical narratives and verbal citation practices as well as non-verbalized facial expressions, gestures, and emotions. Practices are situated and contingent, and this includes the location and whether the activity takes place in homes, cafes, restaurants, or thresholds and entryways to apartments. This can be extended to the importance of bodily and social openings, for instance, the ways people continue to cover and monitor their mouths and noses, or how the transcendental permeates the immanent as belief and possibilities, ranging from the altar to the Virgin in Rosa's restaurant and Maria's belief in political candidates who promised a better future. These boundaries, whether physical or metaphysical, are created and sustained by practices whose tangibility and efficacy can filter and selectively allow things (bodies, materials, images) to enter or exit.

Conclusion: Making pandemic imaginaries and subjects

This chapter has proposed that bodies and practices act as containers and connectors during pandemic change in terms of their ability to both sustain sociality during flux and do so in a way that makes certain images and beliefs compelling or real. What moved many Americans, both literally and metaphorically, during the pandemic crisis was not an empirical notion of what was true or false but what could be made real in their lives through experiential and affective means. With the varied events of the pandemic, uncertainty or rupture was created between peoples' terrain, subjectivity, and wider social movements. Even within a group of people who held the virus to be real, there were different ways in which beliefs were attached to actions and how imaginaries of justice and safety were negotiated through practices. Throughout, questions of boundaries and how one could shape one's landscape were being navigated.

As pandemic subjects, people responded to their newly acquired aware-ness of breath as artistic, political, and entrepreneurial projects, as well as everyday acts of living and coping to process their fraught relationship with breathing, air, and space. Changing circumstances had caused a height-ened sensitivity to breath, reviving feelings of uncertainty and making the landscape seem unfamiliar. Practices became a way to respond to things, restore a degree of ease with the new environment, as well as anticipate the future. Imaginaries of American politics (as social justice or ways of relat-ing to the government) and spirituality (as faith in a transcendental cause or entity) were invoked for their ability to help sustain as well as change things. Normally an unconscious activity, breath became a way to incor-porate heightened concerns into subjects' bodies as they lived in the cov-idscape. This stress on reality as a phenomenological quality of subjects in dialog with social structures helped frame bodies and materials as resources of world-making that shaped relationships between images, objects, and subjects and render future possibilities.

Against the backdrop of a covidscape of pandemic interruption and uncertainty, the complex and varied experiences of COVID-19 survivors and mask stitchers were explored in this chapter through narratives of sick-ness, death, job loss, political upheaval, and changes in daily practices. By using pause and pivot as ways of thinking about breath, practices, and the effects of pandemic interruption, this chapter provided an overview of how Americans responded to the pandemic even as they were in the midst of it. Peoples' uneasiness and tenuous hold on routines and rhythms were appar-ent as documents of flux and adaptation. Various interlocuters' experiences formed a mirror-image to an otherwise invisible virus that could only be known, for most, by its effects and disruptions, lasting long after the actual event of sickness. Conversely, peoples' transformation into certain kinds of pandemic subjects became apparent through their practices and the ways they coped with disruption.

Practices can be framed as generative, embodied ways of coping where pre-COVID-19 concepts of what was an appropriate boundary or distance had to be re-evaluated and earlier imagery brought into dialog with new ones. The levels at which pandemic narratives were shared involved processes of the psychological, phenomenological, and praxeological. The foundational idea of body as container was integral to these varied narratives and indicated how resources of imagination could range from tangible materials and media to reified mental processes and images. Within narratives of bodily change, survivors' experiences included long-lasting sensory effects of the virus on taste, smell, sensitivity, etc. revealing that breath could be damaging as well as rehabilitating, and connecting as well as separating. When bodies were changed by the virus, the effects were unpredictable. For instance, during a moment of panic, experienced in a store's parking lot, Isabel realized that she simply could not continue doing things the way she had earlier. One might say, this was a subjectivating moment where she recognized that she had been transformed.

Belief-making as a way to connect to certain imaginaries and contain (oneself from) others helped bridge gaps between pandemic pause and pivot as the movement between the present and aspirations for the future. Michael and Sarah's imaginary of social justice was entangled not simply with their mask-making endeavors but their experiences of society and the spaces afforded to them as well as changing events. In the case of Isabel, the issue of belief was not a political one but connected with ritualistic aspects of daily practices and her overriding concern with saving her family. Her tactile habits around handling and cleaning groceries separated the sacred from the profane by keeping contagion away—literally leaving it in the passageway. In this sense, the door to her apartment was similar to the airway as a transitional space. For restaurant owners, Rosa and Maria, New York city's mandates on seating in public spaces also became ways of maintaining boundaries and filtering realms. Indeed, they created their own barriers inside the restaurant by placing tables between themselves and customers to create safe zones and ensure the (at that time) mandatory six feet of social distancing. Put together this array of practices and beliefs separated spaces and formed terrains within a covidscape where individual bodies were related to social bodies through entities as diverse as altars, elevators, cemeteries, domestic and work areas, and, ultimately, neighborhoods.

Notes

1 What Goodman (1978) initially explored as the relation of worlds to language and literature, and what is related in this book to actual practices. Many other worlds can exist and we know them as symbolic systems as well as tangible actions and motions.

2 For instance, the CDC permitted the use of two layered masks based on the assumption that the subject was infected and/or asymptomatic. The WHO on

the other hand advised that people use a mask with three layers at minimum. See "Advice on the use of masks in the context of COVID-19," June 2020, p. 9. https://apps.who.int/iris/handle/10665/332293, last accessed 19 March 2021.

3 Douglas (1966: 122) notes that each culture has its own risks and problems, but all "margins" are dangerous ranging from bodily orifices to architectural openings.

4 https://www.wsj.com/articles/new-york-businesses-do-the-pandemic-pivot-to -survive-11586872800.

5 See conversation with artist Cannupa Hanska Luger in the 8 October 2020 webinar, Shaping the Past, by Monument Lab. https://www.youtube.com/watch?v =uFU2UTyQPlE, last accessed 19 March 2021.

6 See Garwood (2011, Section 4, Para. 3).

7 Name is anonymized.

8 Name is anonymized.

9 See Bjork-James (2021) for the powerful hegemonic role and importance of the family in white Evangelical communities in the U.S., and the way this supports rightwing politics and racial segregation.

10 https://forward.ny.gov/cluster-action-initiative, last accessed 21 March 2021.

11 https://nypost.com/tag/vaccines/, last accessed 9 February 2021.

12 https://www.bbc.com/news/world-asia-china-55996728, last accessed 9 February 2021.

13 See Classen (1997, 2012), Howes (2006) and Manning (2020).

14 All names are anonymized.

References

Anderson, B. (1991). *Imagined Communities: Reflections on the Origin and Spread of Nationalism*. London: Verso.

Appadurai, A. (1990). "Disjuncture and Difference in the Global Cultural Economy." *Public Culture*, 2(1): 1–24.

Appadurai, A. (1996). *Modernity at Large: Cultural Dimensions of Globalization*. Minnesota: University of Minnesota Press.

Barrett, L. F., Mesquita, B., Ochsner, K. N. and Gross, J. J. (2007). "The Experience of Emotion." *Annual Review of Psychology*, 58: 373–403.

Bertrand, R. (2021). "Chronicles of a Moral War: Ascetic Subjectivation and Formation of the Javanese State." In U. Mohan and L. Douny eds., *The Material Subject: Rethinking Bodies and Objects in Motion*, 121–134. London: Routledge.

Bourdieu, P. (1977). *Outline of a Theory of Practice*. Cambridge: Cambridge University Press.

Bjork-James, S. (2021). *The Divine Institution: White Evangelicalism's Politics of the Family*. New Brunswick: Rutgers University Press.

Classen, C. (1997). "Foundations for an Anthropology of the Senses." *International Social Science Journal*, 49(153): 401–412.

Classen, C. (2012). *The Deepest Sense: A Cultural History of Touch*. Champaign: University of Illinois Press.

Csordas, T. (1997). *The Sacred Self: A Cultural Phenomenology of Charismatic Healing*. Berkeley: University of California Press.

Csordas, T. ed. (1994). *Embodiment and Experience: The Existential Ground of Culture and Self.* Cambridge: Cambridge University Press.

Damasio, A. (1994). *Descartes' Error: Emotion, Reason, and the Human Brain.* New York: G.P. Putnam's Sons.

De Certeau, M. (1987). *Histoire et psychoanalyse entre science et fiction* [Kindle version]. Retrieved from Amazon.com.

Douglas, M. (1966). *Purity and Danger: An Analysis of Concepts of Pollution and Taboo.* London: Routledge and Kegan Paul.

Du Bois, W. E. B. (1915). "African Roots of War." *Atlantic Monthly*, 115(5): 707–714.

Garwood, P. (2011). "Rites of Passage." In T. Insoll ed., *The Oxford Handbook of the Archaeology of Ritual and Religion.* https://doi.org/10.1093/oxfordhb /9780199232444.013.0019.

Gibson, J. J. (1979). *The Ecological Approach to Visual Perception.* New York: Psychology Press.

Goodman, N. (1978). *Ways of Worldmaking.* Hassocks: The Harvester Press.

Howes, D. (2006). "Scent, Sound and Synaesthesia: Intersensoriality and Material Culture Theory." In C. Tilley, W. Keane, S. Kuechler, M. Rowlands, and P. Spyer eds., *Handbook of Material Culture*, 161–172. London: Sage.

Kearney, R. (2021). "What Happened to Touch?" In A. J. B. Hampton ed., *Pandemic, Ecology and Theology: Perspectives on Covid-19*, 29–40. London: Routledge.

Kemper, T. D. ed. (1990). *Research Agendas in the Sociology of Emotions.* New York: State University of New York Press.

Le Breton, D. (2017). *Sensing the World: An Anthropology of the Senses.* London: Bloomsbury.

Lupton, D. (2013). "Risk and Emotion: Towards an Alternative Theoretical Perspective." *Health, Risk & Society*, 15(8): 634–647.

Lupton, D., Southerton, C., Clark, M. and Watson, A. (2021). *The Face Mask in COVID Times.* Berlin: De Gruyter.

Manning, E. (2020). "Not at a Distance: On Touch, Synaesthesia and Other Ways of Knowing." In C. Nirta, D. Mandic, A. Pavoni and A. Philippopoulos-Mihalopoulos eds., *Touch*, 147–194. London: University of Westminster Press.

Merleau-Ponty, M. (2012/1945). *Phenomenology of Perception.* London: Routledge.

Mohan, U. (2016). "From Prayer Beads to the Mechanical Counter: The Negotiation of Chanting Practices Within a Hindu Group." *Archives de Sciences Sociales des Religions*, 174(174): 191–212.

Morgan, D. (2007). "Seeing in Public: America as Imagined Community." In *The Lure of Images: A History of Religion and Visual Media in America*, 165–195; 282–296. London and New York: Routledge.

Nyamnjoh, H. and Rowlands, M. (2013). "Do You Eat Achu Here? Nurturing as a Way of Life in the Cameroon Diaspora." *Critical African Studies*, 5(3): 140–152.

Perry, S. L., Whitehead, A. L. and Grubbs, J. B. (2020). "Culture Wars and COVID-19 Conduct: Christian Nationalism, Religiosity, and Americans' Behavior During the Coronavirus Pandemic." *Journal for the Scientific Study of Religion*, 59(3): 405–416.

Rozin, P., Remick, A. and Fischler, C. (2011). "Broad Themes of Difference between French and Americans in Attitudes to Food and Other Life Domains: Personal Versus Communal Values, Quantity Versus Quality, and Comforts Versus Joys." *Frontiers in Psychology*, 2: 1–9.

Salpeteur, M. and Warnier, J.-P. (2013). "Looking for the Effects of Bodily Organs and Substances Through Vernacular Public Autopsy in Cameroon." *Critical African Studies*, 5(3): 153–174.

Scheer, M. (2012). "Are Emotions a Kind of Practice (and Is That What Makes Them Have a History)? A Bourdieuian Approach to Understanding Emotion." *History & Theory*, 51(2): 193–220.

Timpka, T. and Nyce, J. M. (2021). "Face Mask Use During the COVID-19 Pandemic—The Significance of Culture and the Symbolic Meaning of Behavior." *Annals of Epidemiology*, 59: 1–4.

Wallace, J. (2020). "Masking: Response-Ability, in Unsteady, Broken Breaths." *Philosophy & Rhetoric*, 53(3): 336–343.

Warnier, J.-P. (2006). "Inside and Outside: Surfaces and Containers." In C. Tilley, W. Keane, S. Küchler, M. Rowlands and P. Spyer eds., *Handbook of Material Culture*, 186–195. London: Sage.

Warnier, J.-P. (2007). *The Pot-King: The Body and Technologies of Power*. Leiden: Brill.

Whorton, J. C. (1982). *Crusaders for Fitness: The History of American Health Reformers*. Princeton: Princeton University Press.

World Health Organization. (2020). Advice on the Use of Masks in the Context of COVID-19: Interim Guidance, 5 June 2020. https://apps.who.int/iris/handle/10665/332293.

2 Sewing cloth masks and making do with uncertainty

Introduction

Practices are both socially and technically efficacious (Lemonnier ed. 1993; Mauss 2006/1935). Part of the social efficacy of techniques is reconciling the contingency of images. Through their design, art, and craftsmanship, makers respond to needs as well as anticipating them. By identifying and contextualizing a particular need as a problem and providing a solution, makers of cloth masks help lay paths of connectivity to future possibilities. This future orientation is central to thinking about the potential of exploratory design practices, such as experimentation, prototyping, and reflective critique (Miller 2018: 61). These processes can be regarded as movements of shifting and coping in response to new situations that shape stitchers as specific kinds of ma(s)king subjects.

Activities of making demonstrate similar attitudes toward the world through a belief in humans' power to learn, innovate, and transform (Ingold 2013; Marchand 2012; Sennett 2008). The term "maker" is used here to explore how people evaluate, adapt, and prise out solutions to difficult problems by leveraging things. As such, the 20 or so people I interviewed over 2020–2021 chose to associate themselves with their roles, for instance, as artists, as instructors, as roles in costume shops, or as small business owners. While noting the fluidity and ambiguity of the term "maker" (Marotta 2020), making in costuming alludes both to skilled actions and care in sewing garments and the relationship developed between the maker, clothing, and the person who wears it. That is, making connotes a type of social and material intimacy, connecting body and mind, producers and consumers, categories such as the handmade and the natural, skill and material properties, and embodied and emotional relations with the material world (Carr and Gibson 2016). As part of their roles, costumers, designers, and artists are used to working with inadequate information and filling in the "blanks" where needed. For instance,

DOI: 10.4324/9781003244103-3

a patternmaker has to search online for actors' images and assess fit from photos and the basics of height and weight measurements (Galioto in Jaen et al. 2020: 82). As a process of tinkering or bricolage (Lévi-Strauss 1966/1962: 30), precipitated by pandemic uncertainty, makers use abductive reasoning as they experiment, develop prototypes, and test ideas. In doing so, they manifest Merleau-Ponty's[1] notion of gearing or grasping as taking hold of life as well as acting as "wayfarers" (Ingold 2010: S126), navigating their way through the world and responding to the possibilities afforded by their milieu.

Making do with science and data

By late 2020, masks were widely available and had become ubiquitous in Americans' lives. With N95 respirators being sequestered for medical and healthcare professionals, the lay public continued to rely on washable fabric masks intended as a public health protocol for collective protection. American culture changed to accommodate new safety practices and language due to COVID-19 and part of that was the way emotive images and values were attached to the virus. For instance, healthcare professionals and COVID-19 survivors were referred to as fighters while, depending on one's beliefs, one could be a hero and patriot by wearing or not wearing a mask. Mask compliance over 2020–2022 varied greatly by neighborhood, county, state, and the felt-immediacy of the need. Similar patterns were seen with vaccination rates in the U.S., and masks were entangled within a larger culture of debate and mistrust.

Interviews with mask makers, some of whom are mentioned in this chapter (Sarah,[2] Vinnie, Ashley, Ronn, and Winnie), indicated a section of the population that thought about masks in a sustained manner as well as being a means of exploring how pre-existing practices were attached to masks and adapted. In some ways, makers were as susceptible to the knowledge gaps of the covidscape. This included being part of the lay public and accessing the same scientific conclusions and health policy advice as well as being restricted in material inventory. Feelings of concern, fear, and anxiety around viral spread data indicated that the uncertainty was not just a cognitive entity but a social one. Makers bridged the information gap through their skills and training as well as relying on emotions and feelings (Damasio 1994: 191; Anderson 2006: 749) as desires and processes of risk calculation and decision-making. In exploring makers' states and practices through notions of making do and problem solving, one can explore the kinds of imaginaries makers engaged with, and how bodily states and techniques dialoged with making processes. The manner in which lives became synonymous with mask making is summed up in what Sarah, a theatrical costumer in North Carolina, termed as "survival instinct." When the show that Sarah was working on closed abruptly in March 2020, she was unsure,

> struggling with feeling that I should make a mask but not knowing what would be best or if it is worse to wear a mask. I put out a question on Facebook... A lot of the responses were not positive and it was conflicting, and from the perspective of disposable masks versus reusing masks.

Since disposable masks were not easily available at that time, Sarah decided that "having a cloth mask is better than not having a mask at all."

U.S. makers were concerned about mandates, protocols, and political divisions between organizations. They made their own investigations but were simultaneously very much embedded (even when critical) in the culture of North American healthcare. That is, there was a kind of double consciousness, both trusting the need for governmental control of the situation and struggling with, and recognizing, that the guidance given was inadequate and confusing.

As such, one could say that they were biomedical subjects (Joralemon 2017: 68), operating within frameworks of national and international health guidance and desires. The World Health Organization (WHO 2020) advised that people use a mask with three layers at minimum but the Centers for Disease Control and Prevention (CDC) recommended two or more layers, indicating that advice varied across these two organizations—a pattern that would be sustained through the pandemic. In hindsight it is possible to analyze the two organizations as catering to very different audiences, as well as see that CDC guidance, as minimal as it was, had been watered down or bolstered depending on the state and town. Both the WHO and CDC agreed that "source control" was the main reason for wearing face coverings but erred in saying that the virus was not airborne based on definitions of an aerosol being any infectious particle smaller than 5 μm in diameter, and a droplet being anything bigger. An investigation later showed (Randall et al. 2021) that this was based on incorrect information and that particles larger than 5 μm stayed afloat and behaved like aerosols. The CDC only began to use words like "airborne" or "aerosol" to describe transmission much later, in October 2020, and, finally, in early May 2021, made changes to its COVID-19 guidance, placing the inhalation of aerosols at the top of its list of how the virus spread. These kinds of mistakes, time lags, and the images generated caused a lot of confusion for the lay public.

Since scientific papers were not intended to serve as sources for cloth mask making, when makers tried to supplement the gaps in their knowledge by reading them, there was the problem of a lack of precision on what constituted "cloth." Filtration efficacy numbers of the various kinds of materials used for masks were often cited in scientific and government reports without the required details about the fabric to be used such as thread count and type of weave. This frustrated makers who were anxious about these types of decisions and worried that their masks might make the difference between life and death. In this sense, makers had to do a lot of aesthetic, psychological, and emotive work to bridge the gap between the attainable yet partial efficacy of cloth masks (Balachandar et al. 2020: 14)[3] and the "gold standard" of N95 masks. One might say makers' efforts in interpreting and contextualizing scientific conclusions were a response to the pre-existing problem of "boundary work" by scientists (Nowotny et al. 2001: 57) where science fails to recognize its role in the production of social knowledge.

In a subsequent study that is quite unique for addressing mask makers, a well-made fabric mask is "a three-layer mask consisting of two outer layers of a very flexible, tightly woven fabric and an inner layer consisting of a material designed to filter out particles" (Pan et al. 2021: 730). This is based on studies of CDC mask recommendations as well as the scientists' own detailed specifications for fabrics, aimed at making a recommendation for home sewers.[4] In translating such concerns into a design principle, making a mask became a problem of balancing the type of cloth, say, a 100% cotton with a tight weave, and the number of layers to get the best filtration without too much air resistance. While none of my interlocutors cited mask filtration rates or specific scientific studies, they did speak in terms of material choices, for instance, using words such as "quilter's cotton" or "batik cloth" to indicate sources of tightly woven cotton. Common stories of making do with supply chain issues included reusing bed sheets which have the advantage of being both very high thread count and soft from wear, and using the elastic from lingerie and hair bands. Makers were also clear that the inclusion of multiple layers of fabric as well as a filter enhanced the masks' efficacy although not all of them implemented this in their pattern. These kinds of decisions were examples of a mentality of what was viable rather than what was ideal, bridging gaps between different types of knowledge discourse and what could be realized in an artifact. In this sense, making became a way of dealing with flux by including images from trade, science, and news and social media.

One of the iconic images of the pandemic is, of course, the COVID-19 virion itself. A poster encountered at a plant nursery in Summer 2020 was printed from an image (Figure 2.1) that went viral on the internet. Created by Ander Alencar, a Brazilian graphic designer[5] in March 2020 to influence people to stay home, the image was circulated globally and grabbed peoples' imagination with its rendering of an empty cityscape taken over by red

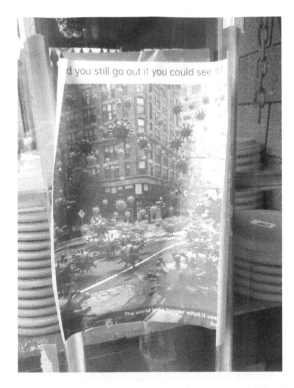

Figure 2.1 "Would you still go out if you could see it?" A popular image of the coronavirus in a plant nursery. Brooklyn, New York. May 2020. Photo by author.

spherical forms representing virions. In reality, the virus is far too small for us to perceive its color: scientists look at it using electrons rather than light, and since light is an essential ingredient in color perception, this means that the virus through the electron microscope exists only in gray-scale monochrome. However, public health campaigns and artistic responses to the virus depict brilliant bursts of color—magenta and orange, velvet blue, deep volcanic red. These colored images are powerful communication tools, but they can also be frightening or, conversely, reassuring depending on the audience.

In June 2020, the WHO released an overview of the kinds of materials to be used and two main types of mask shapes (flat fold/pleated or duckbill), designed to fit closely over the nose, cheeks, and chin of the wearer. While fit was paramount, official guidance by the CDC only came later in a February 2021 report,[6] a year after the pandemic. To avoid opening or shifting during speaking, the shape of the mask had to accommodate facial movements, ensuring that the edges stayed close to the face and could be held in place with elastic bands or ties. Much of this had already been reasoned out on a practical level by makers during the process of sewing. In addition, makers were able to anticipate needs based on what they saw around them without waiting for these to be officially validated. In this sense, makers developed their own space and goals, where images of protection were passed through the filter of problem solving.

Widespread masking revealed needs for people with allergies, face sensitivities, and autism, for those with arthritis or who could not lift their arms, or for masks that could be worn during conversation, singing, or playing a wind instrument. One sewer even made a larger, cup-style, with a clear insert for easy viewing of the wearer's mouth for someone who worked in retail and served many hearing-impaired customers. As terms such as "mask fatigue" and "ear fatigue" came into circulation with the widespread use of masks, users continued to search for the pattern that suited their faces the best. Photos circulated on the internet showing people fashioning their own "ear savers" out of paper clips or plastic bread bag clips; makers came up with variations for this as well through crocheted headbands with buttons, and small elastic strips with buttons that could be used to hold the ends of the earloops. Adjustable ear loops with beads on the ends were introduced later. Gender and age were also considerations when sizing masks to suit the dimensions of faces of children, women, and men, including those with beards. Unique fabric patterns met the needs of specific college and professional teams and young children, especially those who would otherwise refuse to wear masks.

While scientists and health policy makers reinforced the message that the virus was real, for the public, there was a gap between scientific conclusions, mandates, and the affective power of social structures and forms that enabled daily practices. Beliefs that masks are unnecessary or make one sick were manifested in peoples' behavior. When workers in retail and services tried to implement safety protocols, the conflicts that resulted in some parts of the country prompted the CDC to issue guidance, creating a strange situation where epidemiological advice was combined with strategies on workplace violence avoidance. While most businesses had signs put up to inform customers about the need to mask, one store in Omaha, Nebraska,[7] chose to do so in a way that acted as both strategy and commentary, harnessing the logic of an American's right *not* to do something. That "you have a right not to wear a mask. But just like you, businesses have a right to not let you in, not serve you. You can't have it both ways. You are free to make a choice." Here the business was both trying to address would-be patriots, warning them not to "mistake inconvenience for oppression' while also defining what kind of practices were accepted within the store. In doing so, it invoked the mythicized rights of the American subject as individual, albeit "folded" (Deleuze 1988: 94) upon itself.

In response to my queries regarding debates about the usefulness of science, Monona Rossol,[8] an industrial hygienist, noted that science is not about belief but is "a strategy or approach to find the truth based on data." She cautioned that political and economic interests could influence how certain scientific points were emphasized over others but that science itself did not change. Rather it was data that changed and, consequently, the interpretations of that data, as scientists "have to see objectively, quantify and prove up their conclusions." Simultaneously, American science reporters and health and policy experts found themselves in a position where cautious language and caveats were dismissed or regarded as nefarious, unable to reconcile the contingent nature of scientific conclusions with the public's need for immediacy and certainty. They shared how "facts don't change people's feelings. ... You need to understand the beliefs and values that have informed people's reluctance [to health practices]"[9] and that "we have to emotionally evolve with being more comfortable with not knowing things. Misinformation spreads because we don't have a good way to cope with uncertainty."[10]

The human desire for certitude during the pandemic is itself part of, or a response to, modernity where Americans have grown uncomfortable with uncertainty; this is even as social and political change seems more frequently based on emotional valence than reasoned argument. Much like one acquires techniques and attitudes that are suitable for a practice in a given social context, the changing "social life of context" (Dilley 2002: 439) and the act of making (dis)connections are parts of how people are challenged to imagine risk and alter thresholds of the viable, tolerable, and practicable. Here, efficacy is "something to be discovered, cultivated, nurtured, activated and reactivated to different degrees of potency through relationships with others, things and humans alike" (Nyamnjoh 2015: 10).

Creating structure out of contingency

On one hand, human faces were familiar entities for makers but on the other hand there was such variation that the mechanics of fitting fabric to a face was a daunting challenge. Makers worked iteratively, focusing on fit and user experience by tweaking the pattern, dimensions, and materials. Many tested out masks on themselves and chose a pattern that fit their needs and, by extension, also the needs of others. Feedback from users spurred processes of experimentation to generate new mask patterns and refine existing ones to make the masking experience more comfortable. U.S. mask sewing and pattern development projects included those by hospitals whose names were subsequently attached to certain designs, for example, Deaconess,[11] which refers to a type of pleated mask promoted by the hospital in Evansville, Indiana, Florida[12] or a cup-shaped mask developed by a professor at the University of Florida, and Olson,[13] developed by UnityPoint Health, Cedar Rapids. These and patterns from various other sources (Kaiser Permanante, Johns Hopkins Medicine) were circulated online, and adapted and used by American stitchers including costumers from the theater industry.

While techniques in traditional societies are strictly governed by rules of how they may be accessed or acquired, in modernity, techniques have become something that can be acquired through education. Following Mauss' (2006/1935: 81) idea of "prestigious imitation," power is implied in the hierarchy of knowledge in terms of who imparts and who receives. Part of the reason why a person follows a particular technique is the confidence felt in those who have authority because they can successfully perform something. For instance, patterns generated by, or advocated by, hospitals were the first to be adopted by makers reasoning that if hospitals used them then they were probably the best. On a related note, theater costume designers and technologists also retained a sense of their abilities as "professionals" with competencies acquired in institutions and training, and the ability to translate and interpret needs. As such, design is a socio-cultural activity and makers used techniques assembled by and for types of social authority. Designed objects become part of techniques of everyday life, shaped by a consciousness of society, pre-prepared movements, and the rules by which emotions and motions are governed. That is, designers both influenced social forms through their objects and were shaped as specific kinds of ma(s)king subjects.

Making as problem solving

While notions of problem solving may be common to art, craft, and design, here I focus on the quintessential use of this concept in design as the identification of a need and the development of a solution. By comparing design to scientific processes, we can understand how they vary in their goals; "science brackets out events…to arrive at the essentials and primary qualities" while design as bricolage incorporates contingent events to create an artifact or structure (Louridas 1999: 520). That is, science uses the structure of theories and hypotheses to arrive at results whereas making do creates structure out of constraints and uncertainties.

Design has a role in cultural production as a way of making "sense of things" (Manzini 2015: 35), through qualities, values, and aesthetics. These values include a positive orientation toward change through how things ought to be, informed by designers' desire and ability to make sense of emerging situations. Numerous costume designers invoked the idea of problem solving as a way to deal with what they were experiencing, including those in the public eye. Jeff Whiting, the president of Open Jar Studios, home to the "Broadway Relief Project" that employed costume designers among others, described how people in the live entertainment industry were problem solvers used to dealing with unexpected things. Framing the virus as a problem, and identifying it in the form of the mask, helped give shape to the challenges my interlocutors were facing, and made them feel productive. The common mood was one of incredulity that the situation was real as well as a willingness to use their skills to make something. One maker framed it as feeling much more helpless as well as, simultaneously, much more driven to act, indicating a propensity toward responding to uncertainty.

For Ronn,[14] a senior associate professor of theater in his 50s who lived in Washington state, theater was "all about solving problems with the resources you have." Sewing masks felt "repetitive but familiar" and he listed how his skills from theater were forms of know-how put to use. Using processes from the costume classes that he taught, such as sewing, time management, working with quick deadlines, using lighting and audio for Zoom classes, and skills with the university's 3D printers, Ronn worked in an assembly line with costumers who had already been hired for summer theater production. While being socially distant in the theater, the tasks were divided with one person cutting strings, another tracing patterns, two people cutting fabric, and another two who were stitchers. Ronn and a colleague who had sewing machines at home would take pre-prepared pieces home and stitch them. In addition to making 400 masks in this manner for the university, Ronn printed over 100 surgical mask straps for the local nurses.

The early period of mask making was one of experimentation and adaptation since nobody knew how a protective cloth mask was "supposed" to fit. Peoples' first response was to adapt their experiences with masks in woodshops and dyeing labs, making cloth masks as close to the N95 style masks as possible or envisioning how the form of a plastic chemical respirator could be made in fabric. Ashley, a costume designer, observed,

> There was an interesting lag period at the beginning because…there were so many patterns and contradictory sources and new information coming out—even if you found a pattern that worked for you, you ended up changing it if you paid attention to the information stream.

Things seemed to change on a weekly basis with discussions about the various types of fabrics, home science experiments to discern filtration, and a "rush" on quilter's cotton. Then there was debate about the best kind of filter and how to add pockets for filters, whether it was another layer of fabric, folded paper towels, tissue, soft craft paper, coffee filters, or vacuum cleaner filters. As they read and learned more from news and social media, makers gravitated toward the patterns released by hospitals and websites created by fellow makers, such as freesewing.org. Makers also got their guidance in the form of websites and social media (Facebook, Pinterest, Instagram, and TikTok), online news, and videos from fabric and pattern manufacturers, Joann and McCalls.

From the user's perspective, the efficacy of a mask is not discerned just in terms of filtration rates but as fit, silhouette, and comfort. This is literally known through the skin, as sensations of hot and cold, tight and loose, and depending on the temperature and environment, whether the mask feels stuffy or breathable. To arrive at these desired qualities or feelings, the maker should be able to reverse engineer the making process, developing a sensitivity to these features through their own experiences and perceptions. Prior to the making process and its smooth flow, there may be multiple experiments while identifying and adapting a pattern, and through this the maker acquires other types of knowledge. Vinnie, a 30-year-old costume designer from New York,[15] searched out a more ergonomic mask pattern online due to frustration with the fitted shape masks with seams down the middle as well as the standard pleated masks with a bendable wire at the top to fit to the nose. Both these styles led to his glasses fogging up. "I constantly had to adjust it [the nose wire] from slipping…the fabric was pretty much in my mouth any time I had to speak while masked." Instead, Vinnie used a "3D" pattern that jutted out from the face and stayed in place while speaking, eliminating the need for a wire as the curved top edge fit well around the nose.

Certain moments stand out in the sewing process as observed through video recordings made by Vinnie. In the collage in Figure 2.2, the visual knowledge contained in the grid is translated into the pattern template, and from there into various forms of embodied actions, incorporating the whole body as well as an array of tools. To focus on the grid as the starting point of a visual structure, its power is wielded as part of the resources that make up the (possibilities of the) imaginary, providing a double movement that connects idea and matter, the abstract plan and the tangible result. Adapting Krauss' (1986: 12) analysis of the modernist grid as a space of science *and* spiritualism, the grid—or the mapped surface of the fabric—contains but also hides the tension between different belief systems. Part of a mask's efficacy is that through humans' propensity for problem solving it was capable of bridging cognitive and practical gaps that arose between science's claim to ultimate (even transcendental) authority and the messy, real world consequences of freezing conclusions to act upon them. This gap could not be

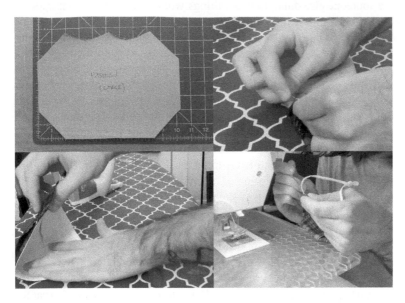

Figure 2.2 The different kinds of skills and knowledge that come together while sewing a mask. January 2021. Photos and video screengrabs courtesy of Vinnie Loucks.

simply fixed by explaining the nature of the scientific process but required effort by the public in accepting practicable solutions embodied by health protocols. As a result, masks do not simply signal belief in the virus or the importance of empiricism (as important as that may be) but the willingness to live with contingency and connect, even if awkwardly, disparate worlds.

To return to the mask-making process, after cutting the fabric for an inner and outer layer according to a template, Vinnie sews the edges of a batch of masks together in one long continuous movement. When turning a sewn mask inside out, he uses a sewing pin to tease out the cloth from a seam and ensure a crisp edge. Such gestures are vital for fit, ensuring that the inner and outer layers of fabric are aligned before further sewing. In the last step, he adds elastic ear loops using a pointed metal tool; introducing a different type of action elastic bits are inserted into seams and then sewn. Much of this work may be attributed to the care that Vinnie demonstrates in making the mask, something we may also identify with the affective side of skill. Vinnie has a graduate degree in costume production, and experience in designing and sewing garments, supplemented by social media. The skills he uses in mask making are those he has used before in other situations, a practice in the sewing world where "we all riff off of each other and things we see someone else doing to make things work best for us." What appears like the smooth and flexible movement of fabric under the sewing machine needle is not just effected by the spatial coordination of the body-and-material but a temporal one, demonstrating knowledge as both memory and a kind of 'instinct' as to what is the next move. The most emblematic tool of this remains the hands through which Vinnie touches the fabric repeatedly to feel whether the inner lining is lying flat and taut (Figure 2.2, lower left-hand corner). He labels this his "perfectionist mind" but this is also part of a "muscular gestalt" (Dreyfus 1972: 249) that responds to situations, adjusting position throughout the making process.

In understanding how Vinnie acquired and enacted these skills and aptitudes, the notion of incorporation of techniques and objects into the subject is useful. That is, objects such as sewing tools, and habits as ways of doing things, are folded into the subject's corporeal schema and body-image, such that the maker is a sewing subject (Schilder 2000; Warnier 2001: 7). Moments of making become unique temporal events drawing on previously acquired knowledge but also performing it in a new context. In Vinnie's words, success at mask making was itself a contingent process, possible for "the time and place I was in" with "skills and tools… [that] worked great for me." The tools and processes he used were also examples of how the past is folded into the present. The chain sewing technique was used to "move things along faster" and came from quilters, the technique with the sewing pins came from handling issues such as small corners on shirt collars, and the metal stiletto—his most frequently used tool and a gift from a friend to help hold down fabric during sewing—was repurposed for inserting ear loop elastic into seams.

From a phenomenological perspective, events project a "double horizon," of the past and future around the present but in the case of the pandemic, movement was also interrupted or brought into question. People experienced a time warp through curtailment of activity and a loss of the hold that one's senses have on temporality as the passage of something. This awareness of not having an optimal grip on the situation created tension, invoked, for instance, in references to "Groundhog Day," the 1993 film in which the same day is relived repeatedly. As a corollary, finding an impetus to make/make-do and move despite the imposed stasis also became a pandemic phenomenon. Searching for "maximum grasp" (Merleau-Ponty 2012/1945: 250) could be regarded as a spatio-temporal phenomenon through which the perceiving body is able to grip objects in space and sense time so that flow is possible. This act of gripping happens literally if one considers how a tool such as the stiletto operates as an extension of the fingers, holding fabric in place as it is fed under the presser foot of a sewing machine. By looking at how these small actions are performed and tools used, the power of grasping as a physical and cognitive technique of "ongoing mastery" (Dreyfus 1972: 162) is revealed.

Making as artistic process

When the pandemic broke, Winnie,[16] a textile artist in her 50s who lives in New York city, moved with her husband and two college-age children back to her previous home in California. I spoke with Winnie on the phone in August 2020 when she had just returned to the city and she reflected on her experience of the early days of the pandemic. Time had "paused" for Winnie and the distinct moments she remembered were in March, November (the elections), and Christmas. She described this condition as "ever March" accompanied by the stress of planning the family's future and her usual role as "resource manager." Winnie also took daily walks, a practice she had sustained for the last 20 years, and decided to undertake a performance art piece on breath and breathing by sewing and wearing a degradable mask on these walks. She sewed some soluble interfacing that she had at home into a mask along with a grid of threads to give it structure. It was 75°F in Northern California and Winnie was curious as to what her breath would do to the fabric.

> It took a couple of days for me to create nose holes. It would harden a little when I took it off. When I put it back on it was a little stiff and I would have to reform it with the breath and mucus. When it started to look creepy is when I started to cover it with a bandana.

Every week Winnie included a reminder of "deliberate manifestation" in her day planner as a way to guide her life's purpose. She had practiced various types of meditation "on and off" and used her stitching art practice to "push" her intention into her work. Winnie documented the mask performance project as a two-week long artwork on her Instagram account under the title "It all fall apart."[17] Each entry was accompanied by the number of steps walked. For instance, the first day was 6 May 2020 and she logged 8,758 steps noting her intent to see how many days or steps it would take for the moisture of her breath to make the mask dissolve. Day 2 was 7 May 2020 and equated 4,992 steps where the dissolving mask continued to shrink as it started to dissolve. "My breath broke through and created two small holes near my nostrils." By 9 May 2020, day 3, 8,156 steps, the "dissolving mask merged with my face (got stuck to my nose." On 14 May 2020, day 4, 8,306 steps, her breath broke a hole at the mouth into the fabric. On 19 May 2020, she documented the last entry of 4,947 steps noting, "I covered my dissolving mask with a bandana—so as not to scare people—as a result I was gasping for air and low key hyperventilating." Satisfied with the results she had achieved and reaching a stage where she could no longer wear the "dissolving mask," Winnie stopped using the mask.

Winnie's experiment with the mask was about breath and transmission as well as a way to cope with how things were changing. The transformation of the mask exteriorized and resonated the changes that she experienced. Enacting control over these changes via the mask helped her respond to the newness of things where information was constantly pouring in about the virus and she had curtailed all activity outside the home except for walking. Appadurai (2004: 81) emphasizes the creative, productive, and generative quality of ritual that is not "the meaningless repetition of set patterns of action, but rather… a flexible formula of performances through which…new states of feeling and connection are created, not just reflected or commemorated." By re-imagining her ritual of walking as a practice of transformative breathing, Winnie tried to investigate what was coming out of her body in the form of breath, moisture, and mucus and how this combination of substances "broke through" the fabric. Walking, during this time, was quite different from simply wearing a functional mask for safe exercise. Winnie was not concerned with the mask's ability to filter virus particles. Quite the opposite, the goal was to investigate the power and efficacy of breath at a time when it had become suspect and was viewed as a vehicle of contagion. Making the mask "fall apart" helped create an artifact that froze the moment and left her with a souvenir of the experience that she could contemplate and share. Echoing words from her own practice, she called the process a "moving meditation" where the material "trapped and immortalized" her breath.

To frame this discussion within problem solving, the maker's skill is based on the ability to perceive as an act of synthesis and motion. While Winnie's exploration did not lead to a functional mask, it did explore the symbolic meaning of functionality through breakdown as well as what it was to ritualize this experiment as daily walks. Part of artists' and designers' training is their capacity to imagine what might be and orient actions toward that image—of creating something by objectifying grasp on the body, on materials, and on the situation. That is, one could regard the ability to respond as coping whether through symbolic exploration of the properties of materials, or making do with changing data and scientific conclusions, the varied stages of public health policy announcements, and lack of material inventory. By bracketing uncertainty and working from a principle or goal, makers are able to assume both a subjunctive and normative position. They enter into a dialog with what is available as ideas, materials, and skills to establish the means to be used, and "integrate internal and external contingencies into a structure" (Louridas 1999: 530). The structure that is developed may simply be a diagram or a sewn grid placed upon soluble interfacing but it enables the making process through which people such as Vinnie and Winnie do things, striving for grasp, and searching for the optimal focus, distance, and point of view. Along with material choices and functions, what goes into the process are cognitive, sensorial, and affective ways of living. How could this observation be applied to other makers and their situational responses to the pandemic? That is, how can the idea of grasp become a way to parse pandemic experience as the ability to obtain something with difficulty, to literally prise something out of life?

The maker as business person

The tensions of trying to grasp and leverage new situations during the pandemic are observed through Sarah's experiences that transformed her from mask maker to business person. Working formerly as a theatrical costumer in North Carolina and with experience in production sewing, she moved in early 2020 from making masks for various local organizations to selling them on the digital commerce site, Etsy. Her virtual store had been established before the pandemic and was hardly used but with theaters closing, and the unemployment check coming in late, Sarah was motivated to activate it to support herself and her family. Through what she describes as the "roller coaster" of her experiences, both in physical retail spaces and the digital space of Etsy, the efficacy of making as coping and cohering can be explored. Problem solving becomes a way to cover both the actions performed on the world and vice versa, or what might be considered as simultaneous objectification and subjectification.

By mid-2021, Sarah had sewn around 3,700 masks and sold most of them via her Etsy store. Her excellent ratings for quality and customer service had become digital markers of her value—her ability to be efficient, source the right fabrics, and create attractive, well-tailored masks (Figure 2.3). But with waning demand around the time that vaccines were first introduced in the U.S. in early 2021, Sarah was "tempering" her expectations for the future since she couldn't possibly make anything that would "go viral" on the same scale as the masks. The word tempering points to not just future orientations and the artifacts that makers produce but the lengthy process of education they undergo through experiences and feelings as a way to respond to life's shocks and jolts (Damasio 2019: 113). Humans' affect machinery is educable as they move, and as argued previously, masks' plenum both literally and metaphorically captures the fluxes of pandemic life. Here air and breath, self and other, internal and external meet and constitute mask makers "as *temperate* (and temperamental) beings… [with] human moods and motivations" (Ingold 2010: S133, emphasis in original).

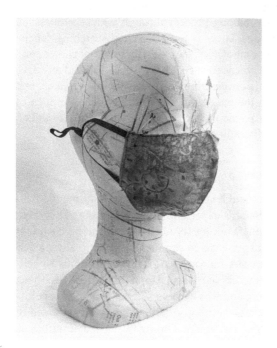

Figure 2.3 A curved pattern mask by Sarah (name anonymized). Image courtesy
of the maker.

Making do and problem solving involve the affective engagement of feelings and social forces. Exploring this engagement indicates how makers are
transformed as they navigate the space between what is ideal and viable,
possible, and practicable.

Drawing upon Sarah's memories, certain key moments in her transformation to business person stand out in the narrative. In one situation at a
bridal alteration store where Sarah worked, she was forced to engage publicly in an unpleasant confrontation with a colleague who refused to mask.
After being made to assert her needs openly in a culture where mask compliance was low, Sarah reflected on the event as one that was framed in
terms of individual rights rather than social responsibility. Much like the
store owner in Nebraska, Sarah was forced to filter her demand that a colleague mask in terms of her rights as an individual rather than being able
to define it as a practice that would benefit everybody in the store. Sarah
continued to follow her own safety practices such as wiping down the sewing machine and reminding customers in the store to wear masks, and these

practices helped solidify her views on the level of risk she was willing to tolerate in her vicinity.

In addition to the physical store, in the virtual realm of Etsy, the stress of going viral twice and receiving a high volume of mask orders had led to different types of friction both between customer and seller, and in the imaginary of the handmade as a space of authenticity. Sarah stated that her clients wanted "something handmade, they like buying things from an individual human. They can feel good about wearing a mask because it also has all of those qualifiers behind it." That is, there was a relationship of trust formed with customers (mostly women) ordering and reordering masks, sometimes for their whole family. The few times she got negative feedback it was about shipping times, something she had no control over. While her own desire to make and sell was partly based on satisfying a genuine need, the reality of running a business and the notion that the customer is always "right" had made her own emotional landscape far more complex.

Desires of selling and purchasing handmade items on Etsy belong to a long history of the politicization of craft (Krugh 2012) and the imaginary of the creative economy (Luckman 2015) as a space of human connection. While Etsy's founder called for sellers to make masks[18] and the company's mission is "Keep Commerce Human,"[19] in practice Etsy had moved away from the term handmade to advertising the "unique and creative."[20] Under this paradigm a diverse range of approaches toward masks could be found. In late 2021, for those who disbelieved in the need for masks but were forced to wear them, "breathable" cheesecloth masks were available on numerous stores on Etsy. Such stores gave form to the uncertainty surrounding the virus (as well as debates on whether one can breathe in a mask) to make what might be termed anti-mask face coverings. These masks were made of fabric that was loosely woven and permeable while being substantial enough to be worn and washed. For example, one store[21] sold masks made with just a layer of cheesecloth, a loosely woven cotton fabric that as several user photos indicate can be easily seen through and will not block droplets containing viruses. This product accrued thousands of sales and hundreds of admirers. Similarly, various other stores sold cheesecloth masks where buyers chose these "excellent quality"[22] masks for their fit that was so comfortable that one could "forget" it was on the face. While the WHO had previously warned that porous materials would not provide sufficient filtration (2020: 9), the success of these masks because of their sheerness indicates that what is an inefficacious or dangerous design for some is highly desirable for others.

Comments on the site indicated that individuals carefully assessed their needs, the kind of activities they or family members were undertaking, and what the prevailing mask rules were for air travel, sports activities, school, grocery stores, outdoor entertainment venues, and work spaces. Issues of sheerness, lighting, and visibility were included with some helpful commenters advising the use of certain colors over others or recommending a double layer over a single layer to hide facial features sufficiently and make the mask "usable" in public. As one customer stated, "I can breathe easily, no one can see through them, and I can laugh to myself as I pretend masks serve a purpose."[23] More strident commenters, self-identified as anti-maskers or mask skeptics, stated that they used these objects as a way to adhere to "tyrannical rules." Aligned with images of freedom and fed by an "infodemic" (Khazan 2020) of conspiracy theories about masks making people sick, the sentiment repeated most often was one of relief whether from claustrophobia and anxiety or the unreasonable demands of travel, education, or the work place.

While Etsy does not ban such blatantly inefficacious masks, its own concerns become apparent through other means. Tools used to help sellers—sharing customer purchase patterns, search terms, and monitoring store opening/closure, and processing and shipping times—seem to be forms of data transparency. Yet, these are also the result of control and are met with hostility when they impact sellers. For instance, a February 2021 policy[24] forced sellers to agree to off-site ads at extra cost to them. On online discussion boards sellers noted that as a publicly traded company Etsy's goal was to increase its profits; that its policy did not account for makers who were satisfied with their position, and, in contrast to Etsy's desires, did not want more traffic, growth, or orders.

If notions of the real are based on maintaining certain schisms and gaps, they can also involve the collapsing and touching of worlds. In Sarah's case the worlds of the artisanal or craft business and capitalism came together, bringing oppositional desires into conflict. Sarah's interactions were influenced not just by customers' purchasing habits but the practices of Etsy's main competitors, for instance, Amazon's offer of free and quick shipping through its Prime membership, influencing what American customers had come to expect from e-commerce. Such exchanges reflected prevailing rules and norms about the culture of the market, and how customers' desires and sellers' capabilities are mediated through exchange. In the virtual realm, the market as an impersonal force collides with the handmade or craft object as a space to connect with another human being over a shared appreciation of the maker. Drawing a contrast with what she knew of the poor working conditions of Amazon warehouse workers, Sarah described her own preferences to sew in a way that factored in "time for a lunch break or to walk my dog," refusing to work through the night just to be able to mail something out in the morning. In this sense, even while being part of Etsy's corporate structure and vision, Sarah drew an important distinction between her store and a "global conglomerate," sustaining her self-image as a small, independent, human entity with limited resources.

Subjectivity involves states of interiority as well as being subjected to something that exercises power, for example, the rules of the marketplace, as well as having a dimension of autonomy where one is the object of one's own actions. It is in acting and being acted upon that one becomes a particular kind of subject. The notion of going viral, for instance, recognizes Sarah's high levels of success through sales. Her work had value not simply due to the store's popularity but the fact that it met a vital, urgent need. But the mode by which such needs were met contained tensions. Sarah certainly drew upon abilities of constant problem solving as a human ability but some of these problems arose precisely because of the space in which she operated. Previously, we had discussed Vinnie's handmade mask as a space that contained diverse images. Similarly, Etsy's handmade goods strategically connected it as a publicly traded company (with capitalistic goals for growth and speed) to the image of the maker-entrepreneur as independent and artisanal. It is in containing and bridging this contradiction, even if temporarily, that we can say makers were subjectivated as pandemic stitchers, gaining knowledge of business practices, and relating changing life and work expectations as a means of transformation.

Conclusion: Making as solving problems and building worlds

Much of the discussion of masks' efficacy is their ability to form permeable or impermeable barriers and to selectively allow entry and exit to breath, moisture, and virus-laden droplets. But in its social role, a mask is a surface that connects as well as contains. The plenum that is contained by the mask can be explored as a space of pandemic flux, where air and breath, and private and public, meet and touch awkwardly with contesting values and beliefs at play. Through the affective side of making do and problem solving, we can see how makers navigate their own goals in the space between what is ideal and viable, possible and practicable, relying on their abilities to evaluate a situation and objectify concerns through practices. The beliefs attached to objects and images exert compelling forces on people in contexts ranging from moral obligations to simply providing or enacting an aesthetic interpretation. All these become ways to categorize the world, shape it, and conclave value as power and potential.

One of the main arguments in this chapter was that through a close look at making, one can explore how homemade cloth masks were recontextualized from objects of idealized efficacy, that is, from things as close to N95 masks as possible to objects that could comply with CDC and WHO recommendations. Further, as masks became objects of daily use they became associated with other imaginaries beyond health, such as political messaging embodied in the cheesecloth mask. That is, through their materials, aesthetics and meanings masks were made to fit with concerns that were not directly connected with epidemiological function. What exactly was a compelling need or problem and how it was to be met depended on makers' specific values and imaginaries. There was variation even within home-made or home sewn masks and the process of deciding what a mask *could* be—in the face of contradictions and gaps—was an example of bricolage thinking and navigating.

Masks do not simply symbolize but are part of a covidscape of science, health practices, and responsible citizenship. When it comes to makers, their confidence to be able to problem-solve could itself be seen as a kind of image that had to be put into action, filtering anxiety and uncertainty especially in the early stages of the pandemic when people did not know if masks were useful or dangerous. The social and symbolic considerations that they engaged with to make these masks—values, beliefs, and recognition of certain forms of authority—emphasized certain techniques over others as non-technical but nonetheless efficacious factors. Through these connections, images and materials needed for worldmaking were deployed, embedding the object (and its maker) in a world of relationships. That is, mask makers could be regarded as containers of knowledge, connecting their problem-solving capacities and bricolage approach with evolving information about the virus.

Problem solving and making during the pandemic emerged as the process of containing tensions and contradictions whether consciously or unconsciously. While certain abilities, skills, and knowledge from pre-pandemic times were used as a starting point to assess needs and identify resources, developing a structure within which to move forward was both literally and metaphorically a unique response. What could be considered a unique situation or event also varied, ranging from Vinnie's adapted motions and gestures of making, to the ways in which these actions sewed together imaginaries of customer needs and business success in the case of Sarah. Problem solving was not the resolution of contradictions but the feeling of completeness via the ability to contain diverging forces and make the world coherent and traversable through practices and productions. That is, problem solving's efficacy was both in the artifactual and in the social domain, framed spatio-temporally by the context, and processes of coping and navigating.

The tensions of trying to grasp and make sense of situations can be explored through Vinnie and Sarah's experiences as processes of subjectivation, transforming them into mask makers. Further, in Sarah's case, making offered changes in situations and perspectives, and the opportunity to shift or change position into a business owner. By encountering new problems and contradictions, these shifts became motions and relationships of coping and navigating. That is, it is in studies of motion that subjects' abilities to prise solutions or grasp life are revealed. When there is stasis, there is no change of situation, context, or interaction, and therefore no way for the subject as event/response to happen. Thus, the making subject is always a moving subject—it is a posture toward and of the world, and material and visual culture is incorporated into the analysis from this position. Makers do not navigate a pre-determined world but make worlds that help contain the uncertainty of the pandemic as well as creating new narratives. That is, the use of bricolage is not just about tackling an inventory of materials but, in the original Lévi-Straussian sense, of connecting ideas and images as myth-making resources. In addition, subjects as bodily-and-material entities leave traces and lay paths of connectivity to future possibilities. Problem solving could thus be seen as a process that relies on feeling, sensing, and imagining the world.

Notes

1 Merleau-Ponty (2012/1945), endnote 47, 496–497.
2 Name anonymized.
3 Thanks to Monona Rossol for sharing this study. The filtration efficiency of cotton masks falls dramatically from that of an N95 between the 0.1 and 10 μm range, and it is that range that mask efficacy must ideally target.
4 If the mask fits well, this approach enables high performance in single-flow inhaling and exhaling modes to produce an overall efficiency of >70% at the most penetrating particle size of .3 μm and >90% for particles 1 μm and larger. In comparison, the CDC non-sewn and CDC sewn mask materials had efficiencies of ~50% at 2 μm.
5 See https://www.instagram.com/p/B-YdqEElj8m/, last accessed 23 July 23 2021.
6 The report (Brooks et al. 2021) was released as part of the CDC's "Morbidity and Mortality Weekly Report" (MMWR) series.
7 https://www.instagram.com/p/CCZesqKJ0eK/, last accessed 16 July 2021.
8 Personal communication with Monona Rossol, 27 November 2020.
9 "The Atlantic's Ed Yong: 2020: Our Pandemic Winter: Darkness, Hope, and Covid-19." 7 December 2020. The Cooper Union. https://www.youtube.com/watch?v=_rgJs2A1fBA, last accessed 8 March 2021.
10 Roxanne Khamsi in "City of Science: Truth and Lies: Covering COVID-19." 24 February 2021. The Graduate Center, CUNY. https://www.youtube.com/watch?v=LsqmRlemSuc, last accessed 8 March 2021.
11 https://www.deaconess.com/How-to-make-a-Face-Mask, last accessed 12 July 2021.The pattern was developed by The Turban Project.
12 https://anest.ufl.edu/clinical-divisions/mask-alternative/#prototype2, last accessed 12 July 2021.

13 https://www.unitypoint.org/cedarrapids/sewing-surgical-masks.aspx,   last accessed 12 July 2021.
14 Interview with Ronn Campbell, 5 August 2020.
15 I am grateful to Vinnie Loucks for sharing his time and expertise with me as well as documenting the process via video and photos.
16 The artist's full name is Winnie van der Rijn and her artworks can be viewed at www.winnievanderrijn.com.
17 The project can be viewed at https://www.instagram.com/p/B_2tU-dlPPw, last accessed 7 February 2021.
18 See "4.7.20 Update: Mobilizing our Community in Times of Need, April 7, 2020," by Josh Silverman, https://blog.etsy.com/news/2020/mobilizing-our -community-in-times-of-need/, last accessed 2 July 2021.
19 https://www.etsy.com/mission, last accessed 20 July 2021.
20 www.etsy.com/about, last accessed 2 July 2021.
21 https://www.etsy.com/shop/thatrockymtnmama, last accessed 3 April 2021.
22 The various comments on these masks were collated from: www.etsy.com/list- ing/827505469, last accessed 3 April 2021.
23 https://www.etsy.com/shop/ShellyNaturals, Comment by Danielle, posted 15 February 2021.
24 https://www.etsy.com/seller-handbook/article/introducing-etsys-risk-free -advertising/729663416588, last accessed 23 July 2021.

References

Anderson, B. (2006). "Becoming and Being Hopeful: Towards a Theory of Affect." *Environment and Planning D: Society and Space*, 24(5): 733–752.
Appadurai, A. (1986). "Introduction: Commodities and the Politics of Value." In A. Appadurai ed., *The Social Life of Things*, 3–63. Cambridge: Cambridge University Press.
Appadurai, A. (2004). "Capacity to Aspire: Culture and the Terms of Recognition." In V. Rao and M. Walton eds., *Culture and Public Action*, 59–84. Stanford: Stanford University Press.
Balachandar, S., Zaleski, S., Soldati, A., Ahmadi, G. and Bourouiba, L. (2020). "Host-to-host Airborne Transmission as a Multiphase Flow Problem for Science- based Social Distance Guidelines." *International Journal of Multiphase Flow*, 132: 1–20.
Brooks, J. T., Beezhold, D. H. and Noti, J. D., et al. (2021). "Maximizing Fit for Cloth and Medical Procedure Masks to Improve Performance and Reduce SARS-CoV-2 Transmission and Exposure, 2021." *Morbidity and Mortality Weekly Report*, 70(7): 254–257. http://doi.org/10.15585/mmwr.mm7007e1.
Carr, C. and Gibson, C. (2016). "Geographies of Making: Rethinking Materials and Skills for Volatile Futures." *Progress in Human Geography*, 40(3): 297–315.
Damasio, A. (1994). *Descartes' Error: Emotion, Reason, and the Human Brain.* New York: G.P. Putnam's Sons.
Damasio, A. (2019). *The Strange Order of Things: Life, Feeling, and the Making of Cultures.* New York: Vintage Books.
Deleuze, G. (1988). *Foucault.* Minneapolis: University of Minnesota Press.

Dilley, R. M. (2002). "The Problem of Context in Social and Cultural Anthropology." *Language and Communication*, 22(4): 437–456.

Dreyfus, H. (1972). *What Computers Can't Do: A Critique of Artificial Reason.* New York: Harper and Row.

Ingold, T. (2010). "Footprints Through the Weather-World: Walking, Breathing, Knowing." *Journal of the Royal Anthropological Institute*, 16(S1): S121–S139.

Ingold, T. (2013). *Making: Anthropology, Archaeology, Art and Architecture.* Oxon: Routledge.

Jaen, R., Durbin, H. P. and Essin, C. (2020). *Theatre Artisans and Their Craft: The Allied Arts Fields.* New York: Routledge.

Joralemon, D. (2017). *Exploring Medical Anthropology.* London and New York: Routledge.

Khazan, O. (2020). "How a Bizarre Claim About Masks Has Lived on for Months." *The Atlantic.* https://www.theatlantic.com/politics/archive/2020/10/can-masks -make-you-sicker/616641/, last accessed 21 June 2021.

Krauss, R. (1986). *The Originality of the Avant-garde and Other Modernist Myths.* Cambridge: MIT Press.

Krugh, M. (2012). "Joy in Labour: The Politicization of Craft from the Arts and Crafts Movement to Etsy." *Canadian Review of American Studies*, 44(2): 281–301.

Lemonnier, P. ed. (1993). *Technological Choices: Transformation in Material Cultures Since the Neolithic.* London: Routledge.

Lévi-Strauss, C. (1966/1962). *The Savage Mind.* London: Weidenfeld and Nicolson.

Luckman, S. (2015). *Craft and the Creative Economy.* New York: Palgrave Macmillan.

Louridas, P. (1999). "Design as Bricolage: Anthropology Meets Design Thinking." *Design Studies*, 20(6): 517–535.

Marchand, T. (2012). "Knowledge in Hand: Explorations of Brain, Hand and Tool." In R. Fardon, O. Harris, T. Marchand, C. Shore, V. Strang, R. Wilson and C. Nuttall eds., *SAGE Handbook of Social Anthropology*, 260–269. London: Sage.

Mauss, M. (2006/1935). "Techniques of the Body." In N. Schlanger ed., *Techniques, Technology and Civilisation*, 77–95. New York: Berghahn Books.

Manzini, E. (2015). *Design, When Everybody Designs: An Introduction to Design for Social Innovation.* Cambridge: MIT Press.

Marotta, S. (2020). "Making Sense of 'Maker': Work, Identity, and Affect in the Maker Movement." *Environment and Planning A: Economy and Space*, 53(4): 638–654.

Merleau-Ponty, M. (2012/1945). *Phenomenology of Perception.* London: Routledge.

Miller, C. (2018). *Design + Anthropology: Converging Pathways in Anthropology and Design.* New York and London: Routledge.

Nowotny, H., Scott, P. and Gibbons, M. (2001). *Re-thinking Science: Knowledge and the Public in an Age of Uncertainty.* Cambridge: Polity.

Nyamnjoh, F. B. (2015). "Amos Tutuola and the Elusiveness of Completeness." *Wiener Zeitschrift für kritische Afrikastudien (Vienna Journal of African Studies)*, 29(15): 1–47.

Pan, J., Harb, C., Leng, W. and Marr, L. C. (2021). "Inward and Outward Effectiveness of Cloth Masks, a Surgical Mask, and a Face Shield." *Aerosol Science and Technology*, 55(6): 718–733. https://doi.org/10.1080/02786826.2021.1890687.

Randall, K., Ewing, E., Thomas, E., Marr, L., Jimenez, J. and Bourouiba, L. (2021). "How Did We Get Here: What Are Droplets and Aerosols and How Far Do They Go? A Historical Perspective on the Transmission of Respiratory Infectious Diseases." *SSRN*. https://papers.ssrn.com/sol3/papers.cfm?abstract_id=3829873.

Schilder, P. (2000). *The Image and Appearance of the Human Body*. Oxon: Routledge.

Sennett, R. (2008). *The Craftsman*. Stanford: Yale University Press.

Warnier, J.-P. (2001). "A Praxeological Approach to Subjectivation in a Material World." *Journal of Material Culture*, 6(1): 5–24.

World Health Organization. (2020). Advice on the Use of Masks in the Context of COVID-19: Interim Guidance, 5 June 2020. https://apps.who.int/iris/handle/10665/332293, last accessed 8 March 2021.

3 Performing care and world-making

Introduction

An exploration of the pause-and-pivot dynamic considers how makers respond and find new ways of containing and connecting via imaginaries and associated practices, values, and beliefs. The events of 2020 heightened awareness that people in the U.S. inhabit divergent spaces in terms of proximity to the effects of the virus. That while simplistic, containment models dominated accounts of viral spread, its trajectory was human-made and could only be understood through sociological complexities (Sugrue 2022: 3). In a stunning illustration of institutional and governmental failure, there was insufficient Personal Protective Equipment (PPE) for "essential workers"[1] when the pandemic first spread in the U.S. Systemic problems, such as broken supply chain systems, increased the number of people who fell through the cracks of social and economic inequity. The issue of which bodies faced risk, such as those of bus drivers or home health care workers, raised concerns over the gendered and racialized nature of essential labor in the U.S. (Lupton et al. 2021: 73) as well as highlighting the "syndemic" nature of the pandemic (Bambra et al. 2021: 3). That is, the pandemic was not only experienced unequally but exacerbated by social, economic, and health inequalities. Against this backdrop of crisis, several grassroots movements were formed (Grayson 2021; Pleyers 2020) to redress inequity and lay Americans, mostly women, felt compelled to sew masks and gowns.

By sewing masks, makers expressed care for their families, friends, neighbors, and strangers. Care is a diverse concept, including caring about something "as an emotion or disposition," caring for something as "a form of labour or physical work," and "care as a social relationship" (Buse et al. 2018: 245). Care can also be connected with subject making in the sense of "care of self" (Foucault 1997), a way of understanding a modern self that is compelled "to face the task of producing" itself (ibid: 311) through "a form of continual self-*bricolage*" (ibid: xxxix, emphasis in original).[2] That is, the

DOI: 10.4324/9781003244103-4

processes of making that we encounter in a world of objects and images include a constant re-making of selves as part of a modern subjectivating process. Further, an important dimension of this process is that it not only shapes the actions and identity of the subject but does so by subjecting it to other people's expectations, demands, constraints, and power. Indeed, questions of identity and politics are very much part of this process when subject making is connected with world-making and the maker wishes to "transfigure" something by taking hold (French: *prendre*) of it or grasping it (Foucault 1997: xxxii). The term "grasp" connotes both the ability to physically hold something and know or understand it on an intimate level. Holding or grasping is also a historically contingent process that avails of the "heterogeneous parts and forms available" (Foucault 1997: xxxvii) at any given moment. Thus, the metaphor and practice of grasping as a subjectivating process invokes both the ability to act and be acted upon. It lends itself to an intersectional analysis[3] of power where makers' hold over the world is a performance with intentionality but is also constrained by structural and institutional forces. In the context of grass roots movements that emerged over 2020, grasping the world through a "resistant imaginary" (May 2015: 12) helped challenge images of labor by asking who did care work and for whom, and focusing on the value of work done by distinct racialized, ethnicized, and gendered bodies.

In this chapter, interviews with members of two sewing groups, Auntie Sewing Squad (ASS) and Broadway Relief Project (BRP), as well as individual mask stitchers help explore how care is part of a group's practice that shapes subjects as relational entities. Further, when sewing practices are regarded as metaphors and techniques of political change, they draw attention to how traditional notions of "craft" intersect with making as empowerment (Alvarez and Fernando 2021: 183) and performance (Butler 1990, 1993; Graeber 2012: 29) to provide alternative images (Collins 2019: 28) of community and belonging. Sewing projects are also varied in whether "community" is an explicit focus of the group wherein community as a term has emotional resonance and evokes "a thick assortment of meanings, presumptions and images" (Amit and Rapport 2002: 13). Some groups/makers have a relatively apolitical desire to support themselves financially while others extend the idea of economic inequity and vulnerability to social justice and volunteer projects where sewing is part of affectively engaged, "core" (Selznick 1992: 184) relationships. By strengthening "ties between the social and symbolic domains of social change" (Collins 2021: 109), for example, care can become a core image in affectively engaged mutual-aid[4] groups.

While all relationships can be considered exchanges ensuring some degree of cooperation, those based on expediency and financial gain alone result in more tenuous bonds predicated on psychological and moral distance. In contrast, core or more intimate participation relies on members being subjectivated as "caring subjects" through engagement with the group's values, reflecting "connections that are central to a person's life experience and identity" (ibid). Despite their differences both these broad models of sociality engage culture as values, routines, and structures. In both cases, the flux of an imaginary has to be felt, known, and negotiated as real via performance.

Performance, politics, and care practices

The Auntie Sewing Squad (ASS) was a mutual-aid group made up of predominantly middle-class Women of Color (WOC) and Queer, Trans, and Non-Binary (QTNB) persons of various ethnicities/races who made masks in allyship with marginalized groups in the U.S. (Hong et al. 2021: 42). Started by Kristina Wong, a performance artist, comedian, and elected representative in Koreatown, Los Angeles, the group officially "retired" on 15 August 2021 after 509 days of existence as a "caring community of Aunties" and having sewn 350,000 masks as a mutual-aid group. The Facebook post[5] in which this notice was shared cited the group's exhaustion and a form of mission creep[6] where it was not "sustainable" to keep sewing masks by request in an "extractive capitalist culture" wherein "the same capitalist systems that fly billionaires into space fail to provide a basic living wage to their employees." In doing so, the squad also drew attention to "the historically undervalued labor of women, especially women of color," noting their surprise at how their "unpaid labor has been requested by well funded non-profits and even government agencies." The group invoked the ideas of kinship and care that lay in the term "Auntie," drawing upon the cultures of its original Asian-American members that were affirmed by the rest of the group. The group's mandate also emphasized how value is associated with certain kinds of labor, leading to social inequities and neglect of minority and marginalized peoples in the U.S.

In October 2021, Wong started performing her pandemic memoir and show "Kristina Wong, Sweatshop Overlord" at the New York Theater Workshop. She opened the show by sitting down at a red Hello Kitty sewing machine whose mechanics had been suitably altered, and "sewed" for a few minutes. The sewing machine and the brightly colored props of boxes and outsized sewing paraphernalia (Figure 3.1) were positioned on a white stage against a wall covered with masks. The stage was designed to reference Wong's studio in Koreatown, Los Angeles, from where she led the squad over 2020–2021. She began her monologue by exclaiming that she was "acting," drawing the audience's attention to how the sewing she was

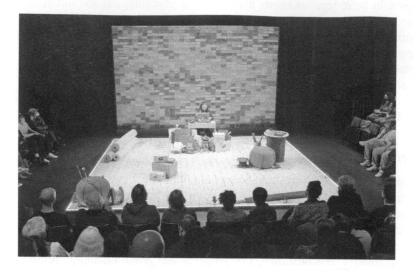

Figure 3.1 View of a performance by Kristina Wong. October 2021. New York. Scenic Design by Junghyun Georgia Lee. Costume Design by Linda Cho. Lighting Design by Amith Chandrashaker. Reproduced with permission from New York Theatre Workshop.

doing was not real and, thereby, pointing out the representative frame of the show. By doing so, she created intimacy with the audience and invited them to co-inhabit this space as a creative interpretation of her experience and pandemic history. Wong's performance of 90 minutes was complex with the personal, social, and political events of two years layered upon each other. To illustrate the passage of time, Wong frequently referred to media images and themes, sometimes projected onto the backdrop behind her. She also pointed out how her own face acted as a "mask," hiding her identity as American and marking her as somebody of Asian origin at a time when the virus was referred to xenophobically as the "Chinese virus." Wong continued framing her experiences and perceptions of the pandemic through an internal dialog and occasional exchange with the audience. Using a combination of drama and comedy, she conveyed how a casual group was transformed into a national, mutual-aid force.

Since most of my interlocuters in this chapter are from the performance world it is worth exploring their notion of the social as a mode of performance. That is, the term "performativity" can be used to analyze the power of practices to shape subjects and effect change in the world. During a Zoom interview in 2020, Wong emphasized the ability of artists to develop something larger out of their ability to make-do.[7] That "it [the pandemic crisis] taps into that thing that artists have when you don't have a lot of resources. You can't afford to go order a costume so you make a costume." While making-do is something I explored in the previous chapter from the perspective of effects on a single person, here Wong described leading the squad as "running a different kind of ensemble theater." That is, the making of ASS as a social justice group with a strong political voice shows how sewing became a subjectivating event that brought together people who would otherwise not be in proximity. In addition, this maker group could be considered as a community of performance that cohered some as insiders and separated others as outsiders by foregrounding certain values and beliefs. The story of Wong's organization and mobilization of a mutual-aid community through sewing is subsequently narrativized and amplified by her theatrical performance.

Self-fashioning practices in Auntie Sewing Squad

The formation of groups during the pandemic reflects how culture has become less of Bourdieu's *habitus* (1977: 72), a tacit realm of reproducible practices and dispositions, and more "an arena for conscious choice, justification, and representation, the latter often to multiple and spatially dislocated audiences" (Appadurai 1996: 44). Naming and citational practices act as boundary markers that divide insiders from outsiders, providing pathways for claims to power. Further, the semiotic and affective excess of names as well as the legal, social, and aesthetic power implied makes them useful organizing tools. For instance, diverse peoples are placed in one group in the U.S. when they are referred to as "Asian Americans and Pacific Islanders" (AAPI). This broad ethnic classification refers to people of East Asia, South Asia, Southeast Asia, the Philippines, and the Pacific Islands, which one might argue does not do justice to the cultural backgrounds of these communities, and yet, despite debate (Kibria 1998), the term "AAPI" remains useful as a means of cohesion and representation within the U.S.

Bodily practices and aesthetics are crucial for generating the affective register that makes it possible for things to be felt and experienced. However, since interviews with makers were conducted primarily via Zoom during the pandemic and, indeed, much of the mask makers' exchanges were through social media, it is also important to focus on these as digital spaces of care. Virtual practices that cohered ASS ranged from online chats and photos on social media to online exercise sessions. Facebook, Twitter, and Instagram were used as a means of organizing and civic engagement when they amplified the lack of masks, helped arrange for supplies, and communicated needs between makers and recipients. One of these early social media incidents also included a confrontation that took place on a global stage. In early-mid 2020, some of the early members of the squad formed a vocal group on the FreeSewing.org site to challenge and contest the name of a mask pattern. Joost De Cock, a stitcher from the Netherlands, who also happened to be the founder of the site, had created a curved mask pattern and named it as "Fu." By challenging the use of this name as being both racist and performative, a small group of articulate squad members were able to get De Cock to change the name of his pattern to "Florence." In addition, they were able to adapt and rename the pattern for their own purposes by calling it UVH after "Uncle" Van Huynh, a "real life Asian."

Comments by squad members in the online discussion thread observed how the power of a name provides for self-definition as a "fundamental human right" and that there has been a "long Orientalist tradition of conflating people from all Asian countries into one anonymous mass."[8] Since Fu wasn't connected to an actual person it perpetuated this stereotype and served as a "casually racist interpretation of what the Chinese (or "Asian") language is."[9] The renaming of the "Fu" mask pattern to UVH was valuable as a critique and mobilizing tool for the squad as it acknowledged a real person's life, and commemorated how he had actually made masks by altering the pattern to make it a better fitting one. In naming the mask pattern as "Fu," even if intended as a form of tribute, the original pattern creator De Cock had relied on a connection with a stereotypical, fictional character, popularized in the West as a style of mustache called the Fu Manchu. The squad's public critique of this name as a form of performative allyship and their subsequent creation of an alternative shows how dominant imaginaries can be successfully resisted.[10]

Yoga practices on Zoom

The pandemic was a return to focusing on the domestic familial unit, the home as stage on which practices took place, and the household as "a site of micro-level social processes that bring together social reproduction, biological reproduction and economic production" (Hawkins 2016: 105). In addition to the physical "pods" that people formed to meet and socialize during the pandemic, virtual pods were created through social media and video conferencing to satisfy needs for connection and well-being. "Auntie" Puneet, an Indian-American "caring" auntie, offered free "calming" Hatha yoga sessions for fellow squad members that they could attend via Zoom while at home. Puneet,[11] a yoga instructor who lived in Los Angeles, California, was in her early 50s. She had dealt with a lung condition since childhood in India and had returned to yoga as an adult in the U.S. with such success that she had weaned herself off medicines. Puneet termed yoga as a "universal" practice, indicating how yoga moved from a

Hindu practice (for instance, Holdrege 2014: 14) to a physical technique or a spiritual practice without doctrinal or institutionalized religious ties that could be practiced by anyone.

Kristina Wong[12] attributed the staying power of the squad to the community they had built wherein "we don't just care for others with our sewing but we care for each other." The terming of certain activities as care begs the question as to what was considered harmful. Since squad members were caring for each other how did they deal with the negative effects of sewing work? While being interviewed over a Zoom meeting, Wong described the physical toll of sewing as she gestured how stress is felt through the curvature of the spine, neck, and through to the hands during the act of sewing on a machine. That is, the typical sewing posture engaged and affected the entire body of the stitcher from the eyes to the feet running the pedal. Puneet's yoga session dealt with the effects of repetitive sewing motions and how "stress" or feelings of emotional and physical tension were "taken" and "held" when stitchers demanded more from their bodies through certain positions such as the rounding of backs, necks, and wrists. She described "taking the outside in" and "moving breath" or *prana*[13] (Sanskrit, which refers both to the energy of one's self and of the universe as life force) to different parts of the body as some of the ways practitioners worked through the adverse effects of stitching. The ways in which she spoke to practitioners helped them control their thoughts as well as guide their motion while focusing their attention on their breathing.[14] Simultaneously, their "body images"[15] were being shaped through their sheer physical proximity to objects, such as yoga mats, blocks and virtual screens, and the social relationships mediated through group yoga sessions.

Through its ability to control the body and mind, yoga can be related to ideas of self-care as a "technology of self" (Foucault 1988). Drawing on a previous study of the "bodily-and-material" (Mohan and Warnier 2017), techniques and affects are means of subjectivation where practices transform peoples' sensori-motricity as well as emotional and psychological states. Puneet's description conveyed how by gaining awareness of their feelings via a consciousness of their posture, and mental and bodily sensations, practitioners developed a felt sense of self (interoception) that, in turn, gave them greater agency and control. Concepts, such as meditation and immunity, formed "themes" around which she created her yoga sessions and helped create a narrative both for the session and a way to connect it with ongoing events and concerns. There was also emotional stress caused due to various events over 2020–2021, ranging from anti-racism protests to the "agitation" due to U.S. presidential elections and the recount process that was activated in some states. *Asanas* or bodily positions could help deal with this to "release" stress, activating the parasympathetic and cognitive systems and calming people. Indeed, a study of online hatha yoga (Brosnan et al. 2021) concludes that this practice is useful as integrative medicine and telehealth to manage a variety of physical and mental health disorders.

To return to Wong's description of the squad as a form of ensemble theater where members non-hierarchically worked together, the repertoire of care practices were as much part of the "performance" as sewing. The two examples explored above—mask-naming practices and Puneet's yoga sessions—indicated how maker spaces create the "real" of care as something that was felt across analog and virtual spaces. A politics of care was enacted via flows of emotions and affects where bodies were "propped" or rather, sensorially and motrically engaged via objects as diverse as sewing machines, yoga blocks, and digital screens. Puneet enacted bodily postures for psychological and physical relief and provided members with ways to perceive and control their bodies. Both processes could be considered as forms of acting and knowing in order for selves and others to more fully, and relationally, grasp the world. For instance, when practitioners became aware of themselves through the moving of *prana* from one body part to another, there was also the implicit understanding that the body could be monitored, transformed, and controlled by paying attention to what was taken in and held, and what could be avoided or released. Yoga, in this case, was not simply a beneficial exercise routine to deal with stress but a way of caring about oneself to be a certain kind of performing subject, prepared to respond to the world.

Revisiting the "social": From the crucible to the calabash

If they are to work under conditions of volunteerism, the members of a sewing group such as ASS must be willing to engage with other members through commonly held values such as care for marginal communities. In doing so, they engage with an imaginary of the social that is intensely affective and ethical through ideas of justice. In Mauss' (1966) notion of the gift, the social is what is at stake in different forms of exchange and is also a way for "mingling" to take place by combining "personalities and things" (Mauss 1990/1950 in Nyamnjoh 2020: 18, 35). The term "melting pot," originally popularized by Israel Zangwill's (1864-1926) play of the same title from 1908, has acquired mythical status as "a political symbol used to strengthen and legitimize the ideology of America as a land of opportunity where race, religion, and national origin should not be barriers to social mobility" (Hirschman 1983: 398). President Theodore Roosevelt stated during a naturalization ceremony that Americans were "children of the crucible," emerging from the melting pot into a "free land" (Webster 1919: 26 in Smith 2012: 395). Along with this imaginary of freedom is the image of the normative picture of the white citizen who traverses the nation aided by hard, meritorious work and manifest destiny. Even in religion, a topic that will be explored in the next chapter, the discourse of White Evangelical Christianity has tended to ignore the U.S.'s racial and economic divides as systemic forms of injustice (Bjork-James 2021: 6–7). For example, in the case of those who protest government subsidized programs, there is the narrative that the recipients of assistance owe their insecurity to "individual choices, in particular, the choice not to work" (Dixon 2018: 62). The image of American freedom has continued to resonate through the decades in debates ranging from civil rights to mask and vaccination mandates during the pandemic. In conversations with diverse Americans during the pandemic, reflections on the perceived failure of the government to provide PPE as well as protests such as Black Lives Matter (BLM) in Summer 2020 drew attention to pre-existing problems ranging from excessive individualism to social inequity and corporate greed.

Histories of community-building and incorporation of non-white citizens into the U.S. national image rely on processes of "ethnicization" in determining their position in a racial hierarchy. My interlocutors of Asian and Latinx backgrounds narrated how they relied on their own community for support or came to realize the limiting effects of class and race in their own lives. Simultaneously, the invention of groups and labels, such as "Asian-American," indicates how pan-ethnic collectivities respond to the shifting need for political power and belonging within the nation. These are not simply externally imposed desires, and designations such as Hispanic, Latinx, Native-American, etc. are constantly being reframed when people from these communities envision and practice belonging and kinship in specific ways.

The conversations below took place via written interviews, Zoom and phone calls, and the rare, face-to-face discussion over 2020–2021. They served as reminders that peoples' pandemic views were in dialog with the "imagined community" of the nation as well as the ability to differentiate the various kinds of "we" that could exist within the U.S. Norman (Norm), a dancer and actor of Filipino and Tahitian ancestry was in his forties, trying to balance living in mainland U.S. with his ties to Hawaii where he was born and raised. Over a lengthy discussion one evening,[16] he observed the effects of class where people like himself lacked the type of elite contacts needed to advance in their theater careers as well as the interdependent relationships that were necessary for survival. Norm pointed to Polynesian culture where kinship extended to non-blood family through the calabash— usually a large serving bowl made from wood rather than a gourd. One could be a "calabash cousin" by eating from the same container of *poi* (a mashed, starchy food) and, in addition, any woman could be referred to as an aunt or a grandmother where a term of kinship also became an honorific, but implied relational ties.

In keeping with an intersectional approach to care, we can approach containers as images for various social processes: in one instance, people are nourished and linked through commensality as an act that reinforces sociality (Kerner and Chou 2015) and, in the other case, via Roosevelt's image of the American nation, people themselves are melted and digested, made exceptional by the fact of their rebirth. When people faced job loss and food insecurity during the pandemic, this notion of freedom and exceptionalism was brought into question through their inability to satisfy basic needs. In a highly visible illustration of the food scarcity problem, communal fridges began to appear on pavements in various parts of New York City over 2020. Simultaneously, larger programs such as the pantry in Queens Museum, Corona, New York, were started. In collaboration with the civic groups "La Jornada" and "Together We Can," the museum had hosted a weekly food distribution program that began in June 2020. Coincidentally named the same as the virus, Corona is a neighborhood in the borough of Queens in New York City that was at the epicenter of the first wave of the COVID-19 pandemic in New York in 2020. It is made up of mostly Hispanic and immigrant communities and experienced some of the highest cases and deaths. Niceli,[17] an educator and artist in her early 30s from Peru, was an employee at the museum and worked closely with these communities. She noted that life was difficult for people, especially undocumented immigrants since in the beginning resources weren't being properly distributed by the state. And that people survived due to "solidarity between neighbors and friends … and strong family values."

When I visited the food pantry at the Queens Museum, Flushing Meadows-Corona Park, in early 2021, the line of people stretched for a mile, winding around one of the museum's side-entrances and into the adjacent park. There was something poignant about the venue with people of varying ages and ethnicities standing in the cold for hours in the vicinity of remnants from the 1964–1965 World's Fair including the iconic Unisphere—a huge globe that served as the symbol of the fair and humankind's achievements. Adults, often accompanied by young children, and carrying bags and trolleys, waited while their pre-obtained vouchers were cross-checked by volunteers. Once they were waved on, they moved quietly from station to station gathering plastic bags of dried goods, fruits, and vegetables (Figure 3.2). Museum staff were assisted by workers, some paid and others who were volunteers, operating in hourly shifts. On that day two different kinds of activities were taking place simultaneously: people helped offload produce from the trucks outside onto stations on the pavement while others moved heavily laden shopping carts from inside the museum to the

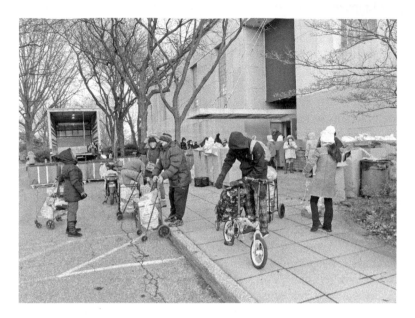

Figure 3.2 Food distribution in progress at Queens Museum. Flushing Meadows-Corona Park, Queens, New York. January 2021. Photo by author.

pavement so that pre-assembled bags of dried food stuffs could be distributed to those waiting in queue. I worked with a group of about five people, mostly Latina women helping hand out the pre-bagged items and gesturing people onto the produce sections where they could collect fruit and vegetables. (The food being handed out was meant to last for a week.) After about an hour of doing this in the cold, I moved into the building where the organizers were headquartered. As I sat at a table that faced a wall and ate a lunch offered by the organizers, a pantry worker sat down some distance away with her own lunch box and struck up a conversation with me. After observing that it was my first day there, she warned me in a friendly tone that, even though I was masked, I was doing it all wrong. Gesturing with her arms outstretched, she told me not to bend over people as I handed out the food. She warned me that the virus was contagious and showed me the stance I should maintain so that I was at the maximum physical distance possible from others.

It was a day of new experiences for me and along with technique advice I was given a slice of the traditional bread "Rosca de Reyes." I was delighted to find a tiny, white, plastic figure of a baby Jesus with his hands and feet frozen in an attitude of prayer. As it was "Dia de Los Reyes" (Three King's

Day or Epiphany), some of the pantry workers in the room, including the drivers who had brought the produce truck to the museum, reminded me that I would have to host a party and cook *tamales* on "Dia de la Candelaria" (Candlemas). But, even as we joked, volunteers continued working in the background, reminding me that this was a celebration that took place against a backdrop of hardship and necessity.

The food pantry envisioned community as a commons of participation and distribution, an idea that resonated in my discussions with some mask makers. Michael, the Chicano designer living in Chicago, had introduced me to Lisa,[18] a Latina seamstress in San Antonio, Texas, in her 40s, who owned a custom dressmaking and sewing studio in a low income and primarily Latinx/Mexican neighborhood. Michael observed that at the height of the pandemic she was still taking client work but also sewing hundreds of masks and giving them away for free. That she felt "compelled" to do this work to save her community and that there is a "very real dynamic and pull that exists between underrepresented peoples and the community that created them." When talking to Lisa via a Zoom video chat in late 2020 she moved around her studio which was empty of people but filled with paraphernalia. She recalled her experiences during the summer of 2020 as those of loneliness and depression, broken-up by sewing masks in her studio and handing them out through the window. Her notion of community was very much situated in the physical neighborhood, her upbringing as a bilingual American as well as a strong belief in reciprocity. As we spoke, Lisa gave me a visual tour of her studio and showed me her worktable covered with red appliqued aprons that would be worn by *matachines* dancers to celebrate the Virgin of Guadalupe on her feast day in December. She was confident that her assistance would not be forgotten. The same people she helped would return as customers in the future when they needed a new dress or even home furnishings—a desire that had emerged during the pandemic.

Lisa's point about community and reciprocity was also underlined by Lily Hope,[19] a Tlingit artist of the Raven moiety, T'akdeintaan clan, based in Juneau, Alaska. In her early 40s, Lily was traditionally trained in Chilkat and Ravenstail weaving, and supported her family during the pandemic by making non-functional masks that became sought after art objects by collectors and museums. Spearheading the #WhyAKMasksUp campaign, Lily was emphatic that "most of America is selfish" and not "for the good of all" minded, contrasting this with the way indigenous peoples "have always worked and lived in the mindset of protecting and caring for one another. My family and my closest friends have kept up this mentality through the pandemic." Discussions also turned to those who have been marginalized either in recent or distant history. "Uncle" Van Huynh, a Vietnamese-American in his early 40s, lived in California after serving 26 years in prison for a juvenile conviction. Van worked with the Auntie Sewing Squad for approximately four months from April to August 2020 and had a philosophical view on life, sharing the reality of the world to be "a hostile and cruel place" and how by contrast, the squad became a "home" that sent out care, empathy, and comfort in the form of masks into the world.[20] Badly Licked Bear, a mixed-race[21] performance artist, educator, and mutual-aid organizer, helped with transporting the squad's masks and supplies to the Navajo Nation, and framed being American as a process of distancing and loss where people "made themselves very special people, separated themselves from all of the human beings by this notion of exceptionalism … people immigrate because they wanna be part of that! So … what do you leave behind when you become an American?"

The comments above invoke the flip side of Roosevelt's vision wherein immigrants are made or rather reborn from the crucible as "free" entities. In its original telling, this narrative of reshaping new Americans is deemed both necessary and positive but being American is also revealed to be a process sustained by contested images, one of them being the equation of freedom with disconnection from previous identities and relationships. Another important image that arises from this de-emphasis on society is the emphasis on the individual and self-containment. Badly Licked Bear interprets the image of American freedom as one of loss for immigrant and indigenous Americans in the U.S., hinting at the complexities of belonging, and Van Huynh shares his experience of how the lacuna of being a marginalized American was filled when a mask-making group provided him with community. For my interlocutors, the question of *how* to be connected as Americans when separated and contained by barriers of race, class, ethnicity, immigration status, or former convictions was very much a pertinent one.

Food from the calabash is the Maussian gift that must be accepted and, at some point, be either transmitted to somebody else or directly reciprocated. That is, things must be shared to pass on their *hau* or spirit. A sense of kinship based on eating from the same pot/fridge/pantry is one way to be relational in the U.S. and commensality is certainly not limited to pandemic-induced events. But what the pandemic made more visible was inequity and how community practices, for instance, organized food commons became a way to fill the gap. What care work and practices made visible was a notion of gift exchange that foregrounds cooperation and sharing as "the *presence* of a conception of the social" (Colesworthy 2018: 37, emphasis in original).

Imagining care through labor and sacrifice

People may care differently about things even as they entangle their own desires and practices with those of a group. In an attempt to further deconstruct the process of pivoting during the pandemic, who was expected to do the work of sewing from home either voluntarily or as a paid activity?

Josephine (Jojo), a costume designer in Anaheim, California, in her early 30s had worked through the spring and summer months of 2020 with the Aunty Sewing Squad (Figure 3.3). She explained how she had to balance two modes of making masks, some made for free as well as others that she sold to support herself. I asked Jojo in late 2020[22] whether she still felt the same sense of urgency in making masks for the squad as in the beginning. She replied that while the repetitive act of sewing could in itself be "numbing," her motivation had been eroded more by the way her labor was evaluated by others. She wondered whether people who received her masks through the squad knew the work that went into them and that they were not disposable since repeat orders sometimes came from the same entity. These

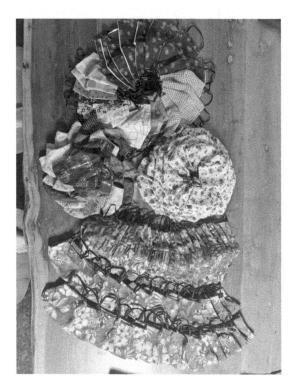

Figure 3.3 A batch of 100 masks sewn for the Auntie Sewing Squad. July 2020. Photo courtesy of Josephine Siu.

experiences, including an encounter with a member of the public via social media, left her pondering how to deal with those "who are just trying to take advantage of the system." That "sometimes people think we will make custom masks for free because we are contributing all these other masks. And that unfortunately makes the urgency [of making masks for free] feel less." Here, Jojo is categorical that although these masks were given away for free to the most deserving they were not providing a "free service."

The affects that compelled stitchers to make were not simply external and were in dialog with complex emotions such as self-evaluations of one's worth tied to income, productivity, and standing in the group. Jojo shared how one colleague who had made an "insane" number of masks was also posting pictures of them on the group's Facebook page. Jojo proceeded to reflect on her conversation with this colleague and how the latter's fear about being removed from the group was acting as a "self-perpetuating pressure." She connected this anxiety to the desire to demonstrate one's productivity, observing how as women "there's never really an end to our to-do list." This left her wondering,

> If I'm not submitting as many masks as the next person, then then what does that say about me? … You know, it's not just about celebrating our work together. It's also about if I don't do this, am I going to feel guilty …

Through her candor and willingness to explore her feelings, Jojo helped relate members' gendered self-esteem to social approval within the maker group, where even if stitchers did not necessarily see or hear from those who received their masks, the value of their labor was recognized through circulation within the group. Simultaneously, it also pointed to how the pressures that makers put upon themselves were part of the process of transforming them as care-givers. When this assessment of self via group approval was disrupted or diverted by a different set of values, for instance, when a member of the public expected masks for free, underlying tensions about occupation and worth were brought to the surface.

The process of being subjectivated and "compelled" to sew through external and internal affects of care is a complex one facilitated by a range of factors. Under conditions of volunteerism, how much makers are willing to sacrifice is connected with feelings of motivation, satisfaction, and recognition (however indirect) gained from helping others. In a conversation between Michael and Jojo in late 2020 about the skills needed to make masks, they emphasized that much of what they did was invisible to people and thus liable to be ignored or devalued. Embedding physical qualities in a mask through its design was also a commentary about *them* as "trained" makers. Their education and skills as designers placed them at a different "level of professionalism" not comparable to just anybody who "dusted off their grandmother's sewing machine" as a pandemic mask maker. According to Jojo, the comfort of a mask and the quality of the cotton and sewing could determine how long somebody would be willing to wear it since "as a costume designer and trained in making I am looking at different details ... a much higher quality than just putting this thing together as quickly as possible." She asked rhetorically, "How are we putting together the seams? Are they straight? ... That's what I'm used to doing in my professional career ... So, when I switched to masks, it was like a smaller version of what we normally do ..." Michael further contextualized this as work "designed for longevity. ... Because what seems superficial like the seams or whether its sewn straight ... add up to create a longer, more durable, lasting product. Our work is never to last just a moment, it's never disposable." While Michael and Jojo regarded these as qualities that were also part of their essence, it speaks to a wider issue of how values are attached to people, and how some people are considered more valuable and others more marginal and therefore more disposable. That is, whether and how the labor value of a specific body shifts when the value of a mask is pegged to its monetary worth.

Gendered values of labor

The topic of industrial sewing in the U.S. and its dependence on the labor of poor immigrant women requires its own study (for instance, Chin 2005) but even stitching by white, middle-class American women took place in 2020 in a climate fraught with tensions around labor and value.[23] Cheri, a retired Associate Professor of Costume Design and Technology based in New Mexico,[24] emphasized the dichotomy of masks both being a desired commodity and undervalued by Americans during the pandemic. Terming it the "ingrained entitlement in American culture," Cheri shared how "one cannot see the discrepancy between urgently wanting to procure masks for oneself (because one has the individual right to protect oneself against a scary pandemic) and demeaning/devaluing the skilled workers who are providing that precious and difficult-to-obtain commodity." She further located this against the general perception of sewing in the U.S. where "no one can imagine what it really takes to create something" as textile production had been outsourced and the measuring stick was cheap, mass-produced garments made overseas.

Eliza,[25] a mask maker from Vermont in her early 30s, noted how mask making intersected with the issue of women's labor and how it was assumed that women who sewed would make masks. While she loved to sew she was also "frustrated" by masks stating,

People wanted my help, and they expected me to donate my time. This felt deeply gendered to me. Sewing, often seen as a domestic skill, somehow lacked monetary value, in the same way that our economy fails to recognize the value of cooking dinner, doing laundry, taking care of kids in the home, etc. It felt as though I should give my time freely, "do my bit" and not expect to be paid.

Robin,[26] a theater designer from New Jersey, concluded that oftentimes women devalued their own work especially writing it off as "nothing." This deprecation was the reason, she argued in a tone of alarm, that masks were selling for just $3 on Etsy. She noted that sewing was not simply something that all women did. "How many women do you know that don't know how to sew? They can't thread the needle!" If a woman could sew, it was not some gendered trait but a valuable, marketable skill.

The felt pressure to sew was echoed in an Instagram post[27] by @ huntersds, dating from the months of March and April 2020. Here, one commenter spoke of the "sense of urgency to make masks" while being "envious" of those who were making quilts (not seen a critical activity at this time) and being "angry" and "perplexed" that others were not helping the pandemic relief "cause." Other women in the same conversation thread spoke of the pressure of expectations—of being "hassled" by neighbors and co-workers to make masks and balancing home tasks with being a "one-woman factory." These social media comments indicate that women were aware of the gendered nuances of pandemic expectations whether invoked within themselves or others, and transparently shared a range of emotional responses as part of a "citational practice" (Goodman et al. 2014) that connected their subjectivity to the wider social, economic, and political aspects of their sewing work.

Broadway Relief Project

According to the website of the Broadway Relief Project (BRP), headquartered at Open Jar Studios, Times Square, New York, the project was "enlisted and approved" by the City of New York and the New York City Economic Development Corporation to make medical gowns for the city's public hospitals. "In 59 days, the project, built over 51,000 gowns, which went directly to the public hospitals of NYC to assist the fight against COVID-19."[28] During an interview, Jeff Whiting, theatrical director and the founder of BRP in New York City, discussed his lack of sewing knowledge when he enlisted the first group of stitchers. Based on a test he determined how fast the job of sewing hospital gowns could be done and created a pay scale based on that speed. But when he sent out the first batch it took the stitchers, who were mostly film, theater, and costume designers, almost twice as long based on the kinds of machines they were using in their homes, the types of materials that could be handled and the size of the gown. The stitchers, also mostly women, were frustrated because the pay per gown seemed very low for the time it took. Jeff noted how "at the end of that first week I was getting nasty emails and phone calls from these people who, you know, we thought in good faith we're doing it right." He had to figure out "what's a more realistic speed and … [how not to] make it slave labor."

While Jeff framed this as his ability to quickly learn and pivot from conditions of "slave labor" to something "realistic" the mode of working remained an industrial or factory-based one. Jessica,[29] a 37-year-old prop artisan, sewed hospital gowns for BRP during the period when film production was closed in 2020. She shared that they were paid $7.50/gown and that payment was on a weekly basis if they completed 30 gowns a week.

> Originally, they had planned for us to complete 40 gowns/week but later they learned that timing was calculated by workers in a professionally set up shop, where tables were made for laying fabric out to pin and the sewing machines were industrial.

If Jessica worked fast she could complete a gown in 30 minutes but her average was closer to 40 minutes. She was slower both because it was taxing on her body and her machine was not industrial.

Jessica shared how a lot of people overused their machines working for BRP or had to figure out different ways of using them. Of her own 2003 machine, since she didn't have a serger or an overlock machine for edging, Jessica came up with her own improvisations, combining fabric rolling with straight and zigzag stitches to finish the seams but this also increased the time. Other things could not be overcome but knowing why they happened helped; an online communal knowledge-base made up of detailed videos of every single step "really helped the people who were maybe kind of lost in the beginning but wanted to stick it out and didn't want to quit." The machine was only going to "go so fast" and the amount of time spent on gowns from one week to the next could vary depending on their size and how seams could be shorter or longer. Jessica's machine worked from the end of April till the last week of May 2020 at which point the main shaft bent. Then she loaned a machine from the repair services to tide her over. It cost her about one week of pay to buy a new machine but the work drew upon people's desire to help in a crisis. That is, the pandemic's ability to evoke sacrifice as the "performance of care" had a ripple effect that extended from people replacing or fixing their machines at their own cost to some repair services loaning out machines for free.

In addition to using her own sewing machine, Jessica would take two buses to the Bay Ridge stop in Brooklyn to meet the van and the drop-off or pickup would take place on the side of the street where, in addition, she could collect anything requested previously such as extra thread or missing/replacement pieces. By not factoring the entire scale of effort both in terms of time spent at the sewing machine and supplementary activities, BRP's calculation of compensation echoed the often "skewed understanding" (Hiltner in Valesky 2020) of the worth of women's labor and sewing work in general. That is, the historical conditions of sewing are important wherein the pre-pandemic costume industry as a whole benefited greatly from the labor and (in)voluntary sacrifice of women stitchers.

Sacrifice implicates the costs and benefits that come with being relationally human and sacrificial value is embodied in the many thousands of masks made by volunteer groups. The *hau* or the spirit of the Maussian gift in these exchanges *is* the image of care that compels connection and return. This return is not simply a transactional one taking place in the course of a one-to-one exchange but can be seen as a form of extended relationality, with the *hau* of care as symbol and practice dispersed through mobilizing networks and opportunities, public recognition, belonging, or companionship. That is, exchanges have effects that extend far beyond and the factors that determine how far these effects will travel can be construed as part of the "social" performance. Care in these relations is not simply a virtue or a latent disposition, but requires practices, for example when the caring subject is created by the relationship between a macro collective politics and a micro ethical and moral relation with the self. Community, as the realization of a social form, is made by common performances based on mutual desires, beliefs, and values. When care is the imaginary that accompanies sacrifice, volunteerism and the sharing of resources become a viable, compelling, and "natural" means of responding to a crisis.

Conclusion: Resistance and alternative worlds

Care is a polyvalent concept ranging from the description of an emotion and disposition to the work of making and sustaining social relationships. Through their repertoire of language, practice, and images, stitchers performed imaginaries of care and turned them into real ways of making their communities. In doing so, they connected emotions with labor and questions of value and belief to form new and different ways of containing and connecting. Performativity was an act with political and narrative significance. It was political in the sense that all actions effect changes in the world depending on their power and there was also an element of story-telling in the manner in which power was imaged and presented. That is, a transformation on multiple levels was necessary to make an imaginary seem self-evident, natural, and compelling. Sewing was a performance and a narrative that cohered people, widening the possibilities of what was considered social, to whom one must feel responsible and with whom one must cooperate.

Intersectionality is important in understanding subjectivation because it emphasizes that power flows and shapes things via the subject who acts in response to others' concerns, hopes, and desires, for instance, as gendered performance of labor. The women in this chapter who are shaped as "care subjects" are also designers and stitchers from the theater and film industry. They live and work in a U.S. theater-scape where womens' worth and sewing work are conflated and perceived as being of less value although this is being challenged increasingly. The perception of gendered labor is also connected to industrial sewing as low-paying, immigrant work and what Cheri, the retired professor of costume design and technology, rues as Americans' inability to *imagine* the work needed to make something. During the pandemic, two major fluxes converge on the issue of inequity—an American melting pot that incorporates immigrants in specific ways and women's gendered worth. How things unfold during the pandemic thus shows how an event can lead to moments where imaginaries expand or contract, hiding the value of labor at some points and revealing it at others. Resistant imaginaries prove useful in helping understand or see the world in a different way. Imagining society as a calabash or food commons is an analogy that can be extended to stitchers as a type of "care commons," providing masks as well as the image that counteracts prevailing imaginaries of the pandemic as one of apathy and loss. For some of my interlocutors, the pandemic also highlighted pre-existing questions of *how* to be connected as Americans when separated by barriers of race, class, and ethnicity. Thus, the metaphor of the container is useful in exploring social processes by which Americans are "stirred" and mixed within the Maussian social while also maintaining boundaries of community and notions of belonging.

The framework of intersectionality helped clarify makers' grasp of the world as the performance of resistance, where transformation—whether of self, others, or the world—was not just a passive act but required an active grasping of an imaginary in the face of fear, threat, and contestation. Performances of resistant imaginaries were very much entangled with care whether it was Michael asserting that his stitching was never disposable or Niceli organizing a food pantry. Care was also exercised through attention to technique where Kristina Wong's attention to bodily posture during sewing echoed the watchfulness of the Latina museum worker who critiqued my manner of handing out food supplies. Both were connected with desires to protect, ranging from a concern with the excessive wear-and-tear on the stitcher's body to how to defend oneself from the virus. As practices, both observations could be considered intersectional ways of doing things, pointing out not just what was to be done but critiquing who was expected to do care work.

While all social relationships involve exchange, the deliberate invocation of emotions, values, and beliefs as well as bonding practices was a variable phenomenon. Auntie Sewing Squad (ASS) and Broadway Relief Project (BRP) used two different models of cohering people to sew. In the squad, stitchers built relational selves and, thereby, involvement around sewing as social justice for certain demographic groups. In BRP, the relationship between stitchers and the organization, while cohered by pandemic urgency, was limited by the monetary compensation model. This is not to say that the squad was free of conflict but that in both these models, varying notions of the social were reflected in the type of community created, and who or what was prioritized.

Notes

1　See Torpey (2020) for details of who would be considered an essential worker.
2　Foucault relates the process of "care of self" to Claude Lévi-Strauss' *bricoleur* (1966/1962: 30) and Charles Baudelaire's (1964) depiction of the modern artist.
3　Crenshaw (1991) and hooks (2006/1994). In framing an "ethics of love" hooks (244) says, "The ability to acknowledge blind spots can emerge only as we expand our concern about politics of domination and our capacity to care about the oppression and exploitation of others."
4　See Kropotkin (1908) for how mutual aid is associated with cooperation as a means of survival among animal and human groups.
5　https://www.facebook.com/auntiesewing/posts/356228916090903, last accessed 4 September 2021.
6　See discussion of mission creep in: Bear, Badly Licked, "Interview with Badly Licked Bear" (2020). Auntie Sewing Squad Interviews. 26. https://digitalcommons.csumb.edu/auntiesewing_interviews/26.
7　For a clip of this interview, see the documentary film "Common Thread" directed by Dorian Coss (2021).
8　See https://gitter.im/freesewing/help?at=5ea479dbafa1f51d4e1da8e6, last accessed on 12 September 2021.
9　See https://gitter.im/freesewing/help?at=5ea47e3e2bf9ef1269a3c0e1, last accessed on 12 September 2021.
10　Of course, the squad's own abbreviated name is a comic reference to "ass"—a performance that invokes attention of a humorous kind.
11　Interview with Puneet Singh Gupta of "Puneet Yoga," 29 September 2021.
12　Interview with Kristina Wong, 18 November 2020.
13　I have chosen not to use diacritical marks for Sanskrit words in this chapter.

14 See Kearney (2008: 267) for how practitioners learn to balance inhalation and exhalation and move from chest-breathing to abdominal-breathing.

15 As Schilder noted (1950/2000: 202) objects in close proximity become part of a human's "body-image," one that "can shrink or expand" by giving parts to the outside world and taking other parts into itself.

16 Interview with Norman Muñoz, 26 July 2021.

17 Interview with Niceli Portugal, 14 January 2021.

18 Interview with Lisa Perello, 22 November 2020.

19 Interview with Lily Hope, 16 August 2020. For more on the artist and her work, see McClain (2021).

20 Interview with Van Huynh, 13 July 2021.

21 They identify as Native American, Latino and Caucasian while being raised by a white identifying Jewish Family who are descendants of Russian and Ukrainian immigrants. See "Interview with Badly Licked Bear" (2020). Auntie Sewing Squad Interviews. 26. https://digitalcommons.csumb.edu/auntiesewing_interviews/26, last accessed 4 September 2021.

22 Interview with Josephine Siu, 3 October 2020.

23 See Pham (2020) for how white, middle class women formed the majority of the civic mask making movements in the U.S.

24 Personal correspondence with Cheri Vasek, 23 March 2021. Cheri worked on over 1,000 gowns for healthcare workers at local hospitals in Santa Fe, New Mexico.

25 Interview with Eliza West, 6 August 2020.

26 Interview with Robin McGee, 19 November 2020.

27 https://www.instagram.com/p/B-tLkLmnRKT, last accessed 25 September 2020.

28 www.broadwayreliefproject.com. In addition to creating PPE for hospitals, the project designed and manufactured masks for singers.

29 Interviews and personal communication with Jessica Smith over 4 August 2020, 24 November 2020, and 27 December 2021.

References

Alvarez, R. and Fernando, A. (2021). "Crafts as the Political: Perspectives on Crafts from Design of the Global South." In D. Wood ed., *Craft is Political*, 181–197. London: Bloomsbury Academic.

Amit, V. and Rapport, N. (2002). *The Trouble with Community: Anthropological Reflections on Movement, Identity and Collectivity*. London: Pluto Press.

Appadurai, A. (1996). *Modernity at Large: Cultural Dimensions of Globalization*. Minnesota: University of Minnesota Press.

Bambra, C., Lynch, J. and Smith, K. E. (2021). *The Unequal Pandemic: COVID-19 and Health Inequalities*. Bristol: Bristol University Press.

Baudelaire, C. (1964). *The Painter of Modern Life and Other Essays*. London: Phaidon.

Bjork-James, S. (2021). *The Divine Institution: White Evangelicalism's Politics of the Family*. New Brunswick: Rutgers University Press.

Bourdieu, P. (1977). *Outline of a Theory of Practice*. Cambridge: Cambridge University Press.

Brosnan, P., Nauphal, M. and Tompson, M. C. (2021). "Acceptability and Feasibility of the Online Delivery of Hatha Yoga: A Systematic Review of the Literature." *Complementary Therapies in Medicine*, 60. https://doi.org/10.1016/j.ctim.2021.102742, last accessed 27 November 2021.

Buse, C., Martin, D. and Nettleton, S. (2018). "Conceptualising 'Materialities of Care': Making Visible Mundane Material Culture in Health and Social Care Contexts." *Sociology of Health and Illness*, 40(2): 243–255.

Butler, J. (1990). *Gender Trouble: Feminism and the Subversion of Identity*. New York: Routledge.

Butler, J. (1993). *Bodies That Matter: On the Discursive Limits of "Sex"*. London: Routledge.

Chin, M. (2005). *Sewing Women: Immigrants and the New York City Garment Industry*. New York: Columbia University Press.

Colesworthy, R. (2018). *Returning the Gift: Modernism and the Thought of Exchange*. Oxford: Oxford University Press.

Collins, P. H. (2019). *Intersectionality as Critical Social Theory*. Durham: Duke University Press.

Coss, D. (2021). *Common Thread* [Video]. Fargofilms.

Crenshaw, K. (1991). "Mapping the Margins: Intersectionality, Identity Politics, and Violence against Women of Color." *Stanford Law Review*, 43(6): 1241–1299.

Dixon, B. A. (2018). "Food Insecurity: Hungry Women." In *Food Justice and Narrative Ethics: Reading Stories for Ethical Awareness and Activism*, 61–76. London: Bloomsbury Academic.

Foucault, M. (1988). "Technologies of the Self." In L. H. Martin ed., *Technologies of the Self: A Seminar with Michel Foucault*, 16–49. Amherst: University of Massachusetts Press.

Foucault, M. (1997). *Ethics, Subjectivity and Truth: Essential Works of Foucault, 1954–1984, Vol. I*. New York: The New Press.

Goodman, J. E., Tomlinson, M. and Richland, J. B. (2014). "Citational Practices: Knowledge, Personhood, and Subjectivity." *Annual Review of Anthropology*, 43(1): 449–463.

Graeber, D. (2012). "The Sword, the Sponge, and the Paradox of Performativity Some Observations on Fate, Luck, Financial Chicanery, and the Limits of Human Knowledge." *Social Analysis*, 56(1): 25–42.

Grayson, D. (2021). "Mutual Aid and Radical Neighborliness." *Soundings: A Journal of Politics and Culture*, 75: 27–31.

Hawkins, H. (2016). *Creativity*. London: Routledge.

Hirschman, C. (1983). "America's Melting Pot Reconsidered." *Annual Review of Sociology*, 9(1): 397–423.

Holdrege, B. (2014). *Bhakti and Embodiment: Fashioning Divine Bodies and Devotional Bodies in Krsna Bhakti*. London and New York: Routledge.

Hong, M. K., Lau, C. Y. and Sharma, P. eds. (2021). *The Auntie Sewing Squad Guide to Mask Making, Radical Care, and Racial Justice*. Oakland: University of California Press.

hooks, bell (2006/1994). "Love as the Practice of Freedom." In *Outlaw Culture: Resisting Representation*, 243–250. New York: Routledge.

Kearney, R. (2008). "Pranayama: Breathing from the Heart." *Religion and the Arts*, 12(1–3): 266–276.

Kerner, S. and Chou, C. (2015). "Introduction." In S. Kerner, C. Chou and M. Warmind eds., *Commensality: From Everyday Food to Feast*, 1–10. London: Bloomsbury.

Kibria, N. (1998). "The Contested Meanings of 'Asian American': Racial Dilemmas in the Contemporary US." *Ethnic and Racial Studies*, 21(5): 939–958.

Kropotkin, P. A. (1908). *Mutual Aid: A Factor of Evolution*. London: Heinemann.

Lévi-Strauss, C. (1966/1962). *The Savage Mind*. London: Weidenfeld and Nicolson.

Lupton, D., Southerton, C., Clark, M. and Watson, A. (2021). *The Face Mask in COVID Times*. Berlin and Boston: De Gruyter.

Mauss, M. (1966). *The Gift: Forms and Functions of Exchange in Archaic Societies*. New York: Norton.

Mauss, M. (1990/1950). *The Gift: The Form and Reason for Exchange in Archaic Societies*. New York: W.W. Norton.

May, V. (2015). *Pursuing Intersectionality, Unsettling Dominant Imaginaries*. New York: Routledge.

McClain, H. (2021). *"We're Still Here": An Interview with Lily Hope*. The Jugaad Project, www.thejugaadproject.pub/home/lily-hope, last accessed 20 March 2022.

Mohan, U. and Warnier, J.-P. (2017). "Marching the Devotional Subject: The Bodily-and-Material Cultures of Religion." *Journal of Material Culture*, 22(4): 369–384.

Nyamnjoh, F. (2020). "Ubuntuism and Africa: Actualised, Misappropriated, Endangered, and Reappraised." *Alternation*, 36: 31–49.

Pham, M. (2020). "'How to Make a Mask': Quarantine Feminism and Global Supply Chains." *Feminist Studies*, 46(2): 316–326. https://doi.org/10.15767/feministstudies.46.2.0316.

Pleyers, G. (2020). "The Pandemic is a Battlefield. Social Movements in the COVID-19 Lockdown." *Journal of Civil Society*, 16(4): 295–312.

Selznick, P. (1992). *The Moral Commonwealth: Social Theory and the Promise of Community*. Berkeley: University of California Press.

Schilder, P. (2000/1950). *The Image and Appearance of the Human Body; Studies in the Constructive Energies of the Psyche*. London: Routledge.

Smith, D. M. (2012). "The American Melting Pot: A National Myth in Public and Popular Discourse." *National Identities*, 14(4): 387–402.

Sugrue, T. J. (2022). "Introduction: Preexisting Conditions." In T. J. Sugrue and C. Zaloom eds., *The Long Year: A 2020 Reader*, 1–14. New York: Columbia University Press.

Torpey, E. (2020). "Essential Work: Employment and Outlook in Occupations That Protect and Provide." Career Outlook, U.S. Bureau of Labor Statistics, https://www.bls.gov/careeroutlook/2020/article/essential-work.htm, last accessed 4 March 2022.

Valesky, M. M. (2020). "Gender Disparity of Women in Theatre Design." *Honors Undergraduate Theses*. https://stars.library.ucf.edu/honorstheses/769, last accessed 18 November 2021.

Webster, H. H. (1919). *Americanization and Citizenship: Lessons in Community and National Ideals for New Americans*. Whitefish: Kessinger.

4 Response-ability and transformation of religious subjects

Introduction

The pandemic unleashed new imaginaries, complicated by death and loss, and schisms in relationships and social forms. Lockdown and "shelter in place" orders took people out of their usual routines and networks of belonging. One way that people addressed these issues was through the care and support offered by religious groups. Faith leaders invoked images of compassion and love as part of collective spirituality and emphasized social connections even as prevailing health protocols called for isolating and maintaining physical distance from others. Still others used this as an opportunity to guide peoples' consciousness in the direction of community engagement as enactment of beliefs and precepts. The differences in faith groups' approaches were apparent when new rhythms and meanings were encountered; some groups were more easily able to adapt to pandemic protocols and health and safety mandates, while others used religion as a means to deny the need for change, for instance, by opposing masking practices and vaccinations. Thus, in responding to the flux of pandemic imaginaries, people's subjectivities shifted and drew upon pre-existing images and objects from religious, political, and governmental spheres as well as creating new connections for interaction and exchange.

Cultures of motricity and materiality[1] are part of practices, generally demarcated in religion as "rituals." While all practices are subjectivating ones in which participants both act on and are acted upon by forms of power, rituals center "a way of acting that is designed and orchestrated to distinguish and privilege what is being done in comparison to other, usually more quotidian, activities" (Bell 1992: 74). However, the line between the ritualistic and non-ritualistic is blurred if we approach them as actions of containing and connecting that flow into and out of faith subjects' bodily and cognitive schemas, influencing experience and perception. From a phenomenological perspective, distance is not necessarily something that

DOI: 10.4324/9781003244103-5

alienates but what makes connection and intimacy possible because it must be traversed, for instance, through contact. That is, distance makes it possible for "things [to] pass into us as well as we into the things" (Merleau-Ponty 1968: 123, in Oliver 2008: 133). Through exchange, whether of breath moving into and out of the body or the movement of objects and images into and out of social groups, pandemic subjects become permeable sites of respiration.[2] One can consider faith groups as "containers," carrying their members' collective "breath" so to speak and whose materially embedded practices act as "openings" (Warnier 2006) for interaction.[3] In previous chapters, examples of such exchange have ranged from the micro-practice of yoga, strengthening mask stitchers' bodies, to the macro-practice of organizing nation-wide sewing efforts. Extending the analogy of breathing as social exchange, faith subjects are shaped through interactions of bodies-and-materials and the ways in which objects and substances, including breath, are (dis)incorporated from subjects (Mohan and Douny eds. 2021; Mohan and Warnier 2017). For instance, a mask bearing an image of the Virgin of Guadalupe (Figure 4.1) is intended for a Mexican or Chicano

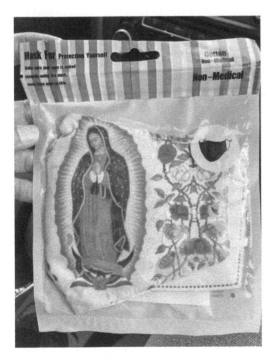

Figure 4.1 A mask with filter bearing the printed image of the Virgin of Guadalupe. Brooklyn, New York. October 2020. Photo by author.

wearer as a kind of Christian subject, invoking the benevolence of the Virgin. Such objects, and the literal and figurative images they bear, are social openings with aesthetic and symbolic value and power. The practices that they engender can be considered as transformative passages, aiding the movement of ideas and substances.

Affects and images of protection and care are embodied in practices through motions such as attaching and detaching, putting on and taking off, opening and closing, and holding onto and letting go. That is, there is a phenomenological and practical "response-ability" between selves and worlds where the Oxford English Dictionary (OED) defines the word responsibility as "a moral obligation to behave correctly towards or in respect of a person or thing."[4] To be relational, faith practices must induce "an obligation not only to respond, but also to respond in a way that opens up rather than closes off the possibility of response by others" (Oliver 2008: 144). Drawing from a phenomenology of experience and perception (Oliver 2008: 133; Wallace 2020: 340), Maussian gift exchange (1966), and the impetus to respond to transcendental other(s) (Reed 2021), responsibility or response-ability is how people engage in exchanges with worldly and otherworldly entities. Within Hindu belief, *dharma* (Sanskrit: individual and cosmic duty, responsibility, rights, laws) invokes an actual way of living where the subject is actively engaged in choosing certain exchanges over others (Mohan 2016, 2019, 2021). In Islam an individual is not self-contained but part of "the networks of belonging that make whole the life of a Muslim self"; this is in stark contrast with the Occidental ideal of the self-determining, self-owning, autonomous individual as the basis of Western liberalism and U.S. Protestantism (Asad 2013: 39 in Strenski 2020; Weber 2001). In an African context, Nyamnjoh (2020: 35) uses Maussian gift exchange to discuss "Ubuntu" as a philosophy of mixing, trust, conviviality, and support.

While the specific entities engaged may vary, this chapter focuses on a few members of two very different faith groups to propose that there is a relationship between faith, exchange, and sociality as response-ability. In doing so, it leads us through two specific practices, the donation of "monk robe fabric" for masks by a Lao Theravada Buddhist temple in California, and a Baptist minister's sermon connecting Christianity with social justice at a Cooperative Baptist Fellowship (CBF) affiliated church in South Carolina. (The CBF is a Baptist denomination founded in 1991 by a group of moderate churches differing from the Southern Baptist Convention over issues such as women's ministry.) In the context of Christianity in the U.S., the minister's approach to pandemic protocols is juxtaposed with some anti-masking voices.

Christian practices and pandemic responses

Many churches used the time of pandemic lockdown to suspend in-person services and encourage their congregation to connect with each other through digital means, using Skype or Zoom for worship. Sacraments, such as communion, were shared virtually,[5] and some priests offered drive-thru confessions.[6] Priests changed their manner of pastoral care and the size of gatherings was reduced with funerals being accompanied only by immediate family. Church leaders asked their members to pay attention to those who were struggling and to help those who were unemployed or sick. Christians discovered new ways to continue to be part of the "body of Christ" and embody his spirit,[7] and pastors asked their congregants to contemplate what their faith meant during this time. While some asked their congregation to think about social justice and the Black Lives Matter (BLM) protests over Summer 2020, other churches responded in ways that reflected their fundamentalist and/or Christian Nationalist approach, demanding that churches be reopened and refusing mask-wearing. Still others within the prosperity gospel tradition offered protection and healing against a "demonic" virus (Stoddart 2021), while a host of preachers offered up a range of conspiracy theories. At the extreme end, were those who regarded the virus as a punishment from God.

Beliefs as sensory, experiential, and emotional states lead people to make connections between certain images while disconnecting and de-emphasizing others. Exploring some different religious subjects produced during the pandemic reveals how spiritual and socio-political images interact in unpredictable ways. For instance, in conversations with a Catholic priest in New York and a Baptist minister in South Carolina, both faith leaders shared stories that were circulating in their communities wherein pre-existing images such as the New World Order[8] and the Book of Revelations' "mark of the beast" were connected with the threat of a COVID-19 vaccine that would insert a controlling micro-chip into people. The readiness of communities that are theologically different to believe in similar ideas pointed to a prevailing national and global imaginary of governance, revealing uncertainty and anxiety about what it was to be "Christian" and "American" during these times.

The culture of the U.S. changed to accommodate new safety practices and language due to COVID-19, and politicizing images and values have been attached to the virus. Over 2020–2021 in daily life and on social media, one could see how affects, emotions, and practices were involved in supporting, resisting, or subverting mask usage or vaccination. For some, defiance and resistance through anti-masking and anti-vaccination related to these practices being not just inconvenient but contrary to ideology and faith, resulting in tense situations. Masking practices quickly became a way to demarcate those whose "religious" commitment was based on the U.S. being "founded as a Christian nation" and the merging of conservative, nationalist policies with divine support.[9] Since the U.S. held a special place in God's plan, the responses and actions of the faithful were divine mandates. Contestation over American rights and freedom moved into an explicitly fundamentalist sphere when harnessed by Christian Nationalists citing Biblical scripture to support anti-masking. In this context, "Christian" does not refer to doctrinal orthodoxy or personal piety but the primacy of beliefs about historical identity, cultural preeminence, and political influence.

An Instagram post by @upscale_for_life tagged with #antimask and #freedomtobreathinjesusname featured a photo of a car's back window with text written on it in white marker. As testimony to the influence of social media on our communication and how "speakers incorporate new technologies of communication from existing communicative repertoires" (Wilson and Peterson 2002: 461), the car window behaved as a "post" of its own—complete with text, a tag line, and a hashtag so that this message was shared with anybody who saw the vehicle go by. The text was from scripture, "The spirit of God has made me; the breath of the almighty gives me life" (Job 33:4). Further, a small U.S. flag, of the size that one could hold in one's hand and wave easily, was attached to the inside of the window, creating a visual and rhetorical intimacy between Christianity, patriotic objects, and anti-masking. Such instances are not isolated and connect trans-medially both with the "imagined community" of the U.S. sustained by print and other forms of mass media (Anderson 1991; Morgan 2007, 2015) as well as the physical presence of anti-maskers. Most protests drew upon both the actions and comments performed at events as well as the power of media to spread their message. For instance, when members of the public defended "God's wonderful breathing system"[10] during the public comment section of a June 2020 Board of County Commissioners meeting, Palm Beach County, Florida, the videos of these encounters went "viral" on social media and news sites.

Depending on desires and demands, the response-ability of people can open up or close off the possibility of responses by others. For instance, during the fluid process of belief-making as navigation of an imaginary, the power of scripture is invoked as one way to establish the "self-evident" nature of one's real. The decontextualized citing of scripture on a car window does not rely on theological knowledge to make its case although it claims that aura. Instead, it relies on multiple other visual and citational contexts (in public townhalls, personal conversations, and social media) as well as its ability to signal something critical—the imagery of breath. During the pandemic, when respiration became a practice of concern, the imagery of breath acquired a greater magnitude both as protection *and* defiance. For example, a consistent and repetitive set of images connect the physical act of human breathing and the transcendental breath of the Almighty (what is called *ruah* in Hebrew) that used to blow at the surface of the oceans at the time the universe was created. For Christian Nationalists, such images, when related to a "sacred" American Union, produce the compelling real that "marches" believers (Mohan and Warnier 2017: 373). The subsequent re-framing of masks and vaccines as a violation of God-given freedoms also draws upon a founding protestant mythology and civil religion (Bellah 1991/1970), where Americans are shaped as "people of the word" and where change is introduced in "the name of continuity, as a return to original principles" (Haselby 2015: 20). For Protestants, the use of pre-existing imaginaries as resources is very much oriented toward a future where they "look ahead for the kingdom to come, pressed there by the intrepid example of the past and nagging uncertainty about the present" (Morgan 2015: 14). The Real of the U.S. as nation thus includes a reverence for the transcendental power of texts ranging from the Bible to the Constitution and, as the examples above indicate, texts become part of practices where belief is "a corporal hexis associated with a linguistic habitus" (Bourdieu 1987 in Rey 2007: 66).

Shifts in Christian subjectivity

For a Christian community, the importance of belonging to the body and spirit of Christ cannot be over-estimated. The faithful Christian not only follows Jesus but joins others in doing so, bearing witness to the covenantal love of God. In this sense faith is relational and social even while being intensely personal.

The contentious response to masking in the U.S. became a prompt for some Christians to understand their relationships with each other as well as how their practices related to theology. In her article on masking (2020), Clare Johnson, an ordained Reverend, mother and wife of a Baptist minister, framed the practice as a Christian one, challenging how those who masked were labeled "sheep." Approaching it from her training as a therapist as well as a faith member, Clare presented masking as a spiritual practice that embodied values of loving one's neighbor, of being humble, of listening, and of remembering that she was loved by a relative or church member who made the masks she wore. Clare's discussion of the mask as something that veiled as well as revealed her as a follower of Christ turned her act of choosing to wear a mask into a declaration of the strength of her bond with God, her neighbors, and her "life of faith."

I contacted Clare via email and interviewed her as well as her husband Matthew Johnson, the pastor of Fernwood Baptist Church, a CBF-affiliated church in Spartanburg, South Carolina. Over a series of Zoom and written interviews, the couple shared how the pandemic had unsettled previously cherished images while providing opportunities to reconsider and identify what mattered to them.

By wearing masks, Matthew and Clare began to experience and notice things that they would not have previously. They described themselves as white, conservative Christians whose lives revolved around family and church and whose ability to fit into a "sweet Southern" community was challenged when they wore masks due to Clare's asthma. Matt narrated how:

> When there was a very low level of compliance as far as mask wearing, when you were the only person in the grocery store wearing a mask, then it very much stood out that I look different. ... everybody else in here is making assumptions about me based on this one thing that I'm wearing and, you know, that's an experience that lot of other people have, but not people that are like us.

In reflecting upon how mask-wearing had affected their relationship with their neighbors and how the practice had "othered" them, the couple pointed to a powerful moment of response-ability. While they could have chosen to ignore this, the couple explored these kinds of moments further, trying to understand themselves and how this impacted their faith.

In answering my question about whether the pandemic had changed how they viewed life, Clare noted that she felt less safe in her country and community knowing that there were so many people who would not be "inconvenienced" to cover their faces to protect her and her family. When she engaged with people who didn't wear masks, the rationale they gave showed they believed in misinformation. She connected the readiness to believe in fake news with the doctrine of inerrancy where the Bible was believed to be infallible and was read literally in terms of history and science. The couple had grown up as Evangelicals and Clare shared that "there is a direct line from inerrancy and authoritarianism in evangelicalism to our current situation in the U.S." Matthew added that all this had made him pessimistic as a minister and self-described "good liberal" who used to believe that people cared about one another, that appeals to reason and "the better angels of our nature" would eventually win the day. Instead, the country's refusal to take COVID-19 seriously indicated deep political and social "dysfunction." Simultaneously, Matthew drew upon what he described as a Christian theology of a "future orientation of hopefulness," acquiring new knowledge that would help him continue sharing his weekly sermons. He upgraded his audio-visual technology and learned how to record and edit videos of sermons so that the congregation could access them regularly.

In June 2020, Matthew delivered a sermon[11] titled "The Fire This Time" while standing in front of the church's stained-glass windows (Figure 4.2). The colorful windows illustrated parables and teachings attributed to Jesus Christ and repeated imagery that the congregation was familiar with, thereby contributing to the worshipful mood. Matthew wore a green stole to mark "Ordinary Time" (Latin: *orior,* meaning to rise, originate, be born), the period between Pentecost, the birth of the church, and Advent, the beginning of a new church year when the birth of Christ is anticipated at Christmas. The sermon took place about a month after the death of George Floyd Jr., a 46-year-old Black man, and Matthew located the death of Floyd, the experiences of Black Americans and the riots in Minneapolis that followed his death within the larger context of the "sin" of racial injustice. He critiqued American society as one that valued "rugged individualism and personal rights" to the neglect of others, manifesting in death and destruction, and imagined COVID-19 as a "fire" that ravaged the most vulnerable populations including people who didn't have the option of working remotely. He also criticized racist interpretation of scripture in the Baptist church where the "Curse of Ham" was used as an excuse to subordinate Black Americans.

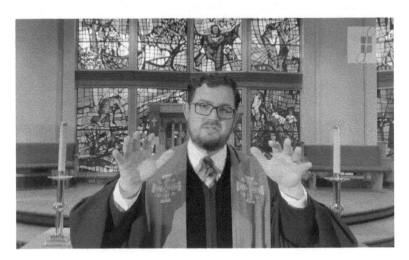

Figure 4.2 "And like flood waters, the infection numbers rise and rise." Rev. Matthew Johnson delivering an online sermon at Fernwood Baptist Church. Spartanburg, South Carolina. 21 June 2020. Video screen capture courtesy of Matthew Johnson.

The "Curse of Ham" comes from the story of Noah's curse upon Ham's son Canaan in Genesis (9: 25–27). Noah curses Canaan into slavery and although Ham is never cursed himself, the so-called "Curse of Ham" has been used to explain the origins of slavery for more than 1,500 years and extended to approve the subservient status of Black Americans based on race. The prevalence of this narrative also relates to the ways in which theology and social privilege intersect in the U.S. and Whiteness acquires a range of transcendental values. That is, it acquires a "mystical," almost "magical" quality (Driscoll 2022: 82), by ignoring the socio-historical processes by which white Christian dominance is asserted.

The renewed attention to bodily safety and protection that arose due to the pandemic extended from the virus to other social and political issues via the issue of governmentality. This meant that faith imaginaries became entangled with practices as diverse as supporting anti-vaccination positions to protesting the teaching of Critical Race Theory in schools. In the covidscape, people discussed, proposed, and contested images of their faith and the American nation based on a transcendental of "democracy, freedom and plenitude" which is "often a re-articulation of (Christian) theological commitments" (Winter 2021). Simultaneously, the pandemic revealed how racism and violence continued in the U.S., for instance, with the police killings of George Floyd, Breonna Taylor, and many other Black Americans.

The results of a Monmouth University Poll (2020) conducted by telephone from 28 May to 1 June 2020 with 807 adults in the U.S. showed that the number of white Americans to say that police are more likely to use excessive force against a Black suspect had risen from 25% in 2016 to 49% in 2020. The poll also found that 76% of Americans said that racial and ethnic discrimination was a big problem in the U.S. Just a few years prior to the pandemic, in 2016, Reverend William Barber II, the then president of the North Carolina state chapter of the National Association for the Advancement of Colored People (NAACP), compared American democracy to a heart that had stopped beating—saying that Americans had to be "moral defibrillators" shocking the nation back to life in the fight for social justice.[12] Indeed, Black voters organized and overcame voter suppression efforts in several key states in the 2020 presidential elections, showing their role in preserving democracy. This was all part of a long history of how nationhood came to be seen as a "medium of divine intention or providence" and where race and religion are "indispensable ingredients of national identity and political self-determination" (Morgan 2015: 165).

Maintaining the right relationship with God in Western Biblical traditions is important as it is connected with "salvation" and draws upon the multiple connotations of the term (Latin: *salus*) including safety, health, wholeness, and deliverance. But salvation is imagined differently when framed as an attitude of defiance of human finitude, expressed when white Americans ignore the state's disciplining of Black and Brown bodies into docility. Matthew's sermon connected salvation with images of spiritual neglect and the possibility of redemption with dynamics of socio-political responsivity. He spoke persuasively to the (virtual) congregation of the connection between the damage and fear wrought by the twin forces of COVID-19 and racism, also placing them within the wider story of Noah's ark (Genesis 6:9) wherein Christians would be left like Noah to set things right and to make the world anew. If the congregation was "surprised" by events such as racism and the protests against masking it was because they had been shut up in their "arks of privilege" while the "storm" raged outside and had not bothered to open up Noah's window—illustrated in the video by the church's stained-glass window—to look out and see what was happening.

The sermon and interviews with Matthew and Clare provided some insight into the couples' view of the pandemic. While his church had not had divisions over closing in-person worship and moving to online worship, Matthew found the process stressful because so much of his work was about building relationships and he could not meet somebody in the hospital or talk over a cup of coffee. He spoke candidly of how preaching a sermon into a camera in an empty room, week after week, had become "emotionally draining." While these effects were in themselves quite negative, the pandemic experience in general was "apocalyptic," a term that means revelation in Greek and that could be translated as an unveiling or unfolding of things. Clare interpreted the word in terms of its moral effects, shocked by the way people protested pandemic protocols, and noting the unsettling amount of "injustice, greed, selfishness, and thick-headedness" in the American population. The theme of unveiling was also a way to understand how faith members understood and responded to pandemic crisis whether it was bolstering their practice of masking or guiding the congregation into what they considered a true, faithful, and contemporaneous interpretation of scripture.

Christianity as a salvation religion leads the individual from one reality to another, setting conditions and rules of behavior that transform the self. Christian rituals such as confession and communion, being specially demarcated, provide members with tangible, shared markers of when and how shifts in religious subjectivation are to take place. Generally, a discussion of Christian subjectivation invokes "technologies of the self" (Foucault 1997: 225) as monastic discipline but is also relatable to the fluidity and indeterminacy of religious imaginaries,[13] each producing its own Real. For example, in the confessional faith of Catholicism, members have a "truth obligation" and must show that they believe with "strict obligations of truth, dogma, and canon" (Foucault 1988: 40). In the context of Baptist faith, the notion of a truth conscience applies even if there is no requirement for a ritualized confession to a priest. For the congregation as well as the pastor, as we have seen in this one instance, the sermon is a means of conveying spiritual knowledge, and providing community and identity to the congregation by connecting different types of images.

Matthew's sermon aimed to elicit a specific kind of awakening or unveiling during the pandemic. It imagined new horizons of relationships as a form of "seeing" that "owes as much to internal imaging as it does to external perception" (Morgan 2015: 135). Although he did not go so far as to frame it in partisan terms, Matthew's interpretation relied on narrativizing scripture in a political manner. There was certainly a concern with naming and thereby addressing the anxiety and fear of the congregation over the unrest and riots that immediately followed George Floyd Jr.'s death in cities such as Minneapolis. There was also the overarching theme of safety, extending from the virus to social and political issues. That is, Matthew tied well-known Biblical imagery of Creation, the presence of the Holy Spirit, and the unfolding of contemporaneous events, binding the individual moral impetus of caring for another human with a wider discussion on race and justice in the U.S. landscape. It was possible to see how faith members might use such imagery to parse their feelings of uneasiness and uncertainty, and stabilize their faith by re-articulating Christian commitments.

Transformation of Lao Buddhist monk robes

Unlike Christianity, soteriology in Buddhism refers to paths of liberation that include those where there is no savior or deliverer to take one there. Spirituality is the aspiration or desire to engage in practices as ways of life that leads one toward the soteriological path and this includes altruistic conduct (Crosby 2014: 12). Merit frequently concerns how an individual relates to or behaves with others, particularly through the lens of charity and morality, and, today, forms of socially engaged Buddhism increasingly focus on this-life solutions.

Traditionally, meritorious action consists of ten actions, the first of which is *dana*[14] (Sanskrit/Pali: generosity, alms) and includes the giving of food, clothing, shelter, and medicine to monks. While food may be given daily, robes are given on specific occasions. *Kathina* or the Buddhist monastic rite of robe investiture is an important merit-making practice in Theravada Buddhism, the oldest school of Buddhism and the dominant religion in Cambodia, Laos, Myanmar, Sri Lanka, and Thailand. Described in the canonical *Vinayapitaka* that regulates monastic life, *kathina's* spread and diversification is evident in Holt's (2017) comparative study of ritual in Sri Lanka and Southeast Asia. That is, while the Pali scriptures of Premodern South Asian Buddhism have lasted for more than two millennia in Sri Lanka and Southeast Asia, even historically, the lived world of the *sangha* or Buddhist monastic community did not coincide precisely with the scriptures[15]. On a contemporary note,[16] when Buddhism from Southeast Asia travels to the West it is reframed variously as "ethnic Buddhism" and/ or "refugee Buddhism" (Ladwig 2017) and there are some changes that take place. For instance, there is a "professionalization of monasticism" (Bankston and Hidalgo 2008: 72) where monks live and stay in the temple serving a de facto congregation. Instead of doing their daily alms rounds in the neighborhood, monks have cooked food brought to them daily. All of this makes these Theravada "forest monks" even more residential and influences the way monks and laity relate to each other. These adaptations can be framed within Theravada temples in the U.S. as "containers" (Cadge 2008: 101, McLellan and White 2005, Warnier 2006) and where the contents they include are a mixture of ethnic origin, migration routes, language, traditions, and the central authenticating role of rituals and ceremonies. That is, the temple provides the community a social form to both connect with its origin country, and redefine itself and engage with prevailing U.S. politics of recognition. Thus, this section traces how Buddhist ritual paraphernalia of monks' robe offerings are embodied spiritual and social "openings" for new kinds of relationships between Lao American donors and non-Buddhist recipients.

In the aftermath of the U.S. "Secret War" and bombing campaign (1964–1975) in Laos, and following the communist Pathet Lao takeover, hundreds of thousands of Laotian refugees, about 10% of the population at the time, fled the country between 1975 and the early 1990s. 90% sought political asylum and United Nations High Commissioner for Refugees (UNHCR) refugee status in Thailand, and eventually resettled in various parts of the world, including the U.S. and Canada.[17] By 2000, a little over one-third of Lao in the U.S. could be found in California where they had established their own Theravada temples. Wat Lao Rattanaram, a Lao Buddhist temple incorporated in 1982, was one of the few temples started with Lao monks who were also refugees themselves and meet the needs of refugees who were resettled in the San Francisco Bay Area in West Oakland, California. Rattanaram refers to the three gems of the Buddha, *dharma/dhamma* (Sanskrit/Pali: righteousness, duty, way of life) and *sangha* (monastic community). The temple moved to its current location in Richmond in 2003, occupying a building that was formerly a Christian Scientist church and in an area that is home to thousands of Laotian war refugees who arrived in the U.S. from 1975 to the early 1990s.

About 15,000 people of Laotian descent live in Richmond and elsewhere in western Contra Costa County. From the web-mapping platform Google Maps, and the temple's Facebook page, it is apparent that the building has been embellished with Buddhist symbols and ornamentation. The site is marked by a flag post bearing a U.S. and Buddhist flag that flies high above a golden wheel of *dhamma* and colorful guardian figures at the entrance. Traces of the building's former purpose are still found in the temple's colorful stained-glass windows although the pews inside were removed and laity sit on carpeted floors. Such temples were, and are, more than religious sites. They help people transition from their previous lives to the "culture shock" of various parts of the U.S. This includes finding employment, dealing with language barriers, and adjusting to new social structures. That is, even three decades later the work of resettling continues and the temple plays a central role.

During the second lockdown in California in January 2021, I started a correspondence with Khammany Mathavongsy, a Lao American in his early 50s and treasurer of Wat Lao Rattanaram. Khammany was dedicated to the Lao American community, to telling its story of resettlement and integration into the U.S., and was a key figure in the political, educational, and cultural recognition[18] of Laotians within the U.S. At the age of 13, Khammany and his elder sister fled to Thailand from Laos leaving their mother and four siblings behind. His father was a Major in the Royal Lao Army and spent 12 years in a Pathet Lao gulag after Laos was taken over by communists. After living for many years in a Lao refugee camp in northeast Thailand, the entire family including his father was resettled in San Francisco. Khammany was also a devout Buddhist and like many young Lao men had been temporarily ordained as a monk in 1991 at the Richmond temple.

Khammany reflected on the initial mood when COVID-19 was perceived as a widespread threat, and the fear, confusion, and lack of information that prevailed. People decided to stay at home over Spring and Summer of 2020, and important temple events such as the annual New Year celebration in April were canceled. The enforced isolation and barriers to interaction also had an effect on the temple's monks who were lonely. Simultaneously, the congregation relied on their faith and on each other (Do 2021). With the statewide lockdown order in California in March 2020, many Lao American women started making cloth masks with different traditional Lao textile patterns. They also made masks out of surplus monks' robes and donated them to different Lao Buddhist temples in Northern California including San Jose, Santa Rosa, Fairfield, Sacramento, and Modesto. While noting that the idea of repurposing robes as masks started *within* the community, I explore how the fabric reached the mutual-aid group called the Auntie Sewing Squad.

Robes as social "openings" between the Lao community and others

The robe ceremony called *kathina* (severe or difficult in Pali; Lao: *thot kathin*, laying down the frame to make robes) takes place once a year after the three months monastic monsoonal retreat, as based on the seasons in Southeast Asia and is a very important event. The following account is based on videos of a *kathina* ceremony in the temple[19] wherein the worship hall is divided into a sacred section for the Buddha figures and monks, and an area where lay people gather and worship.

As the temple's invite for the 2021 *kathina* indicated,[20] the event started in the morning with taking refuge in the three gems, the recitation and observance of precepts, alms offering to the *sangha*, a *dhamma* talk followed by lunch, and the *kathina* robe offering ceremony in the afternoon. The flow of spiritual efficacy was hierarchical, starting from the Buddha figure to the monks as "fields of merit" (Riggs 2017: 201) being seated above the laity on a podium in the temple's main hall. The laity was dressed in their finest with many women and men wearing traditional clothing including silk shoulder cloths *(pa bieng)*. At one point in the afternoon ritual, a string of cotton thread was delivered on a spool by a monk to the laity, one end of which was tied to a robe offering placed on a stand. The other end of the spool was passed to the laity, and both men and women held it between thumbs and forefingers as the leader made his statement of offering. By this time, the thread has been connected to other offerings, including a bed (Lao: *khong kathin*) with items of daily use, such as bedding, utensils, and paper towels, and money trees (Lao: *ton kathin*) festooned with U.S. dollar notes, folded in intricate shapes and used to support the temple's operation. (In a subsequent correspondence, Khammany noted that while the robe was the "heart" of the ceremony, the primary sponsor of the robe offering had shared the merit-making opportunity with others by inviting them to join as co-sponsors.) Once the laity made the offering, the monks received the robes. The thread that connected the robe to the laity was untied and then the robe offering was taken off the first stand and placed on another one. The robes were taken out of their plastic packaging and checked. A small belt with cords on either end was part of the robes and was wound around the set of three cloths. Each end of the cord was wrapped around the middle of a staff with a leaf-shaped fan representing the Bodhi tree under which the Buddha gained enlightenment. The two fans were each held respectively by a monk seated on either side of the offering stand as they recited into microphones. The religious fan de-emphasized the individual monk and thereby stressed that the relationship being created was with the *sangha* as an institution.

A monk's robe is an oblong piece of cloth that is draped, depending on its purpose, as an inner cover/hip wrapper (Pali: *antaravasaka*), chest and shoulder cover (Pali: *uttarasanga*), and outer, double-layered cloak (Pali: *sanghati*). In the past, monks would have sewed their robes out of fabric offered to them by first cutting up the cloth into pieces, destroying its secular value and the possibility of sensual enjoyment, and then using the *kathina* wooden frame to stretch and sew the pieces together. Strict rules defined the making of the robe and, traditionally, this would have been made from multiple pieces of fabric. Strips representing bunds or banks in a rice field, as seen by the Buddha in the kingdom of Magadha, India (Vajirananavarorasa 1973: 15–16), are still used to both order the cloth field and bind it. Today, instead of the monks sewing their own robes, new, ready-made robes consisting of a set of three cloths (Pali: *ticivara*) are gifted by laity. *Kathina* is thus a way for monks and laity to have a Maussian gift exchange, with donations to monks acting like seeds planted in fertile soil, producing a rich crop of merit *(bun)* for the donor.

Rules govern the *kathina* privileges and allowances given to monks regarding ownership or holding of robes. The robe itself acquires spiritual and charismatic value where in some sects of Buddhism it "plants the seed of enlightenment and destroys the poisonous arrows of delusion" (Tanabe 2003: 734). The timing of the *kathina* ceremony after the rainy season is related to both scriptural "connections between the power of the Buddhist monk and agricultural imagery" (Davis 2016: 141–142) and a Lao social life where virtually all ceremonies were timed and held at temples according to the agricultural cycle of seasons for wet-rice farming. Accordingly, monks became fertile fields of merit and as Khammany described it, the gifting of robes was a "small gesture" that had a "big impact." Subjects come to identify themselves with certain objects through a process of ongoing incorporation/disincorporation of object dynamics or material *habitus*. Bourdieu (1977) defines *habitus* through his study of material habituations and dispositions that are continuous and subconscious in a person's life. This is a total process through which the subject and the object are constructed together and for each other and practices are part of subjectivating "coupling" and "decoupling" dynamics. Through *kathina*, laity and monks alternately become gifters and recipients of robes and blessings, establishing a stable and mutual relationship. During the ritual, participants along with the offerings become part of realizing a Lao Buddhist way of life in a diasporic setting, making the faith "real" for the community.

As for the actual outer robe, the use of strips, seams, and the addition of a reinforcing border not only strengthens and binds the fabric but also regulates it. Thread or *sutra/sutta* (Sanskrit/Pali) is a word that lends itself to different contexts including authoritative teachings that are collected or sewn together. Sacred thread (Lao: *sai sin*) is used during rituals to encircle a merit-making group as seen during *kathina*, or to connect individual worshipers with sacred images of the Buddha and monks. In Lao rituals that blend animism and Buddhism, such as *baci,* sacred thread is tied to peoples' wrists to keep mobile souls trapped within a person's body. The Lao believe that each person has 32 spirits (*khuan*) and that under certain circumstances, the spirits could abandon that person, causing sickness or even death. Thus, *baci* is also a way of concentrating the wearer's spiritual force. Also called *sou khuan* in Lao, which means calling back one's soul, *baci* is held at all major rites-of-passage, when a person leaves or returns home, starts a business, or during illness. The use of this practice during pandemic crisis (Do 2021) or historically difficult times, such as Lao refugees' travels to the U.S. (Lee et al. 2012: 26), indicates how thread can be used where there is a need for integration. Apart from the necessary officiating by a monk or elder, the ritual draws upon the properties of thread, that is dynamics of (un) tying and stretching that acquire physical and metaphysical value. That is, the thread becomes a conductor and can be used to make the "charge" flow between spiritual and social realms. This is not just about the objectification of power in objects[21] but, for our purpose, motions by which participants are subjectivated as a Buddhist Lao community. While Buddhist concepts of *anatta* (non-self) and *anicca* (impermanence) prevail, rituals help "fix" the transient bodies of laity (Ngaosyvathn 1990; Van Esterik 1999: 69), giving them a bounded identity.

From robes to masks

In May 2020, the Auntie Sewing Squad received a request for 600 masks from Lao Family Community, an association founded by Laotian refugees in 1980 to help war refugees rebuild their lives. That was a time when the squad was getting national publicity on the news and lots of different people were approaching them asking for masks. In an interview with Ova Saopeng, a Lao American artistic director/producer affiliated with the squad, I learned how a relationship was established between the temple and the squad. Ova described the process as one that started with the squad's founder Kristina Wong wanting to know if this was a legitimate request from his wife, "Auntie" Leilani Chan, a performance artist, artistic director/producer, and cultural worker. Asked by his wife to check with the Lao community if they knew anything about this group, Ova approached his friend Khammany and learned that they were a genuine organization. Like Khammany, Ova's father was a soldier with the Royal Lao Army, who was sent to a re-education camp when the communist Pathet Lao took over the country. Ova's family fled Laos for a refugee camp in Thailand and was subsequently relocated to Hawaii, where Ova and his siblings grew up around other refugees from the wars in Southeast Asia.[22]

Khammany offered to connect Ova with Wat Lao Rattanaram which had a surplus of robes that could be used as mask fabric. He helped arrange for the temple's surplus robes to be given to the squad on two occasions (Figure 4.3). He noted that when those in the temple saw the quality of the "sample" masks made with some of the first batch of robes, they were impressed that it was "professional" and were "even more willing to give more." Ova observed that in some ways, this relationship with the temple "jump-started" the squad's efforts in Northern California bringing in an infusion of fabric, "joy," "blessings," and "excitement." The robes were of various colors, from brown to ochre to orange, with some being pre-sewn or "quilted" from two thin layers—probably *sanghati* or outer cloaks. All were

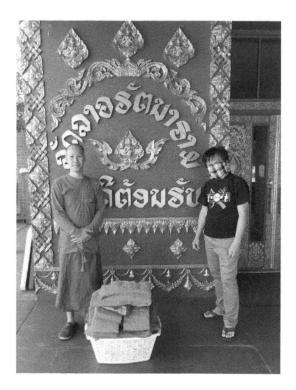

Figure 4.3 Venerable Phra Wistachana Phongadith and Khammany Mathavongsy with monk robes to be donated. Khammany wears a mask made out of traditional checked fabric by a friend. Wat Lao Rattanaram, Richmond, California. July 2020. Photo courtesy of Khammany Mathavongsy and Monica Bullard.

unused and some were brand new. Over Zoom, Ova showed me some of his favorite masks stored in a small box, and commented on how the pre-sewn lines on the fabric became opportunities for his wife Leilani to "play," and respond and stitch the lines into new patterns. Once sewn, some of these masks were sent to a Lao community in Oregon with a note stating what fabric they were made from and requesting that people reuse them. From Facebook comments, it was apparent that masks made with this fabric by other stitchers also went to asylum-seeking families in Texas and Mexico, homeless people in Los Angeles, and protestors in Oakland.

The process of procuring the robes created a map for future activities, developing relationships and establishing a new "node" of the squad so that people could collect and distribute fabric, and orient parcels and sewing pledges. In that sense, the temple and its supply of free fabric were instrumental in helping the squad expand, also creating "solidarity" between BIPOC communities and the squad (Hong et al. eds. 2021: 89). There were two rounds of fabric donation from the temple and "Auntie" Monica Bullard, a quilter, certified nurse-midwife, and legal clerk from Oakland, California, collected the fabric, stuffing the multiple bags into her car and driving them to those who needed fabric. Speaking over the phone, Monica shared how she made about 1,400 masks out of the "monk fabric," sending them to people in Maryland, North Carolina, and Pennsylvania. As a Black American in her 50s, she wore her "protest mask" made with monk fabric to BLM protests in Oakland over Summer 2020, wanting to be part of a "piece of history in the country and part of that voice that was rising up to say this isn't okay, you can't keep killing and hurting us." Monica chose to place the monk fabric on the inside of the mask (paired with her favorite sunflower print on the outside) since it was "special" and where, even if it was invisible, it was "like a blessing," making her feel "safe and warm and cozy." Even among the other Aunties in the Squad, the monk fabric acquired an aura for its "gorgeous saffron" color (Hong et al. eds. 2021: 90), and stitchers were asking for a bit of it to use.

In this chapter's conceptual frame, to be a response-able Lao Buddhist is to be responsive to one's social and spiritual order. Generosity and sharing have an intimate connection with the Buddha's path and the *kathina* ceremony generates merits for the sponsors and receivers. To this list, one may add makers and mask recipients as well. The value of cloth from robe to mask is part of a religious economy of merit cultivated through multiple entities, including the disciplined bodies of monks whose "sacred, immaterial and undying Truth"[23] must be supported by laity. In addition, the effects of these rituals spread widely connecting human and otherworldly entities, helping establish pathways that are simultaneously spatial, spiritual, and social. Only when participants have been integrated and subjectivated within orders of a ritual, a temple, or a nation can they be effective social actors. For Lao refugee communities in the U.S., these orders of containment are not just constraints but vital bonds reintegrating individuals into new settings. Thus, the temple is a center that connects generations in an appreciation of their faith and identity as diaspora in the U.S.

Conclusion: Faith, response, and subjectivation

The faith communities and practices described here are part of a covid-scape—a generative realm of world-making and world navigation. Ways of acting, feeling, and responding become part of the building and contesting of imaginaries where the concept of an "imaginary" does not mean that people necessarily believe in something false or untrue. Rather, it indicates a space of indeterminacy or flux and a capacity to produce images as a sort of compelling reality.

One of the ways religions navigate flux is by drawing upon traditions wherein acting or behaving in a certain way is part of a moral *habitus*. Being social and interacting with one's faith colleagues in a relational manner is expected from others as well as being a framework to act upon and shape oneself as a Christian or Buddhist. The pandemic was a time of re-evaluating pre-existing ways of doing things and adapting old ways by drawing together new images and objects, thereby creating new subjects, new containers, and connections. Faith leaders responded to communities' emotions and states of fear, anxiety, and isolation to guide decisions and responses. The pastor who led the church along with his wife, and the Lao temple's treasurer as well as the monks who sustained the spiritual power of the temple were integral since they exhorted and supported their members in relating to each other—thereby "mixing" the contents of the faith container whether as a temple or church.

Practices of sermons, spiritual ceremonies, and a host of related exchanges, such as sewing, open up new horizons of possibilities by facilitating relationships. For instance, in the case of Laotians, one must consider multiple modes of subjectivation such as UNHCR refugee status that made it possible for people from the country to be ordered within the U.S. as legal entities. That is, religion cannot be separated from other aspects of life that shape the subject and how subjects are shaped, and in turn shape, power flows by choosing to divert, channel, or engage with practices. One can be Christian in various ways as seen in the difference in protocol responses, ranging from nationalist anti-maskers to those who are pro-safety measures. In U.S. nationalist groups, the Christian subject is stridently self-determining, self-owning, and autonomous, made not just by theology but also by the foundational myths of the U.S. such as the establishment of the Constitution, slavery, and immigration laws. The CBF-affiliated church led by Matthew responded to this via a Christian imaginary that connected revelation and awakening to a new horizon of social and racial justice.

How Laotians survive and prosper in the U.S. is not simply an indication of their spiritual strength or their willingness to be "American" but part of a complex response to the types of possibilities available. In a "governmentality of containers" that is the U.S. and where the nation is a power-laden entity, the faithful are subjected to both their own institutions and other peoples' and other institutions' expectations, demands, and constraints as power. Monk robe fabric shaped and smoothened some of these constraints when inserted into new containers of protection and care, in the process blurring boundaries of the secular and spiritual. These relatively flimsy objects also drew attention to how spiritual institutions and leaders helped members negotiate hyphenated identities in the U.S. In the Lao American temple, change and impermanence are to be accepted as constant, framed by the inevitability of Buddhist awakening to life as suffering. But this approach was also accompanied by the knowledge that it was what one *did* after knowing this precept that formed an understanding of reality and, thereby, living in the world.

Notes

1 This adds to the extensive literature on material/sensory religion (for instance, Meyer, Paine and Plate 2010; Morgan 2010, 2021, Promey ed. 2014) from a focus on subjectivation.
2 For more on how breath came to matter in the pandemic, see Lupton et al. (2021: 44-56).
3 As Warnier (2006: 193) notes the process of "passing through" is both a symbolic and literal transformation of contents. Thus, it is worth noting both the ways in which things are passed as well as its representational purpose.
4 See Oxford English Dictionary (2021), www.oed.com/view/Entry/163862, last accessed 22 February 2022.
5 For discussions of "presence" and "ocular communion," see Parish (2020).
6 https://abcn.ws/3bhA2RK, last accessed 10 February 2022.
7 See Reed (2021: 119) for the importance of moving from "representing" Christ to "possessing" him as revelation and spirit, as encountered in the event of the Pentecost.
8 The New World Order is a unifying conspiracy theory found in religious and secular contexts where events are connected with an immensely powerful, secretive group that aims to seize control of the world.
9 See Whitehead and Perry (2020: x).
10 https://www.bbc.com/news/av/world-us-canada-53174415, last accessed 4 February 2022.
11 The Fire This Time, Genesis 6:9-14; 18-19; 8:8-12; 9:8-17, Fernwood Baptist Church, 21 June 2020. https://vimeo.com/431019617, last accessed 6 February 2022.

12 http://www.cnn.com/TRANSCRIPTS/1607/28/se.02.html, last accessed 30 January 2022. Thanks to Tamar Samir from drawing this to my attention.
13 See Mohan and Warnier (2017: 374).
14 I have chosen not to use diacritical marks for Sanskrit, Pali, and Lao words in this chapter.
15 See Collins (1997: 48).
16 See Bankston and Hidalgo (2008), Cadge (2008), and Van Esterik (1992, 1999).
17 See Lee (2015: 146–149) for more on this subject.
18 He was also a Founding Board Member for the Center for Laos Studies and a Board Member of the Bay Area Lao Association. See De Voe (2008) on the role of Lao community leaders in bridging the gap with wider American society.
19 For videos of the *kathina* ceremony, visit https://www.facebook.com/watlaor attanaramrichmond/videos/.
20 https://www.facebook.com/watlaorattanaramrichmond/posts/ 1565227543825222, last accessed 27 February 2022.
21 See Tambiah (2013: 327) on ritual objects as "sedimentation of power."
22 https://anotherwarmemorial.com/ova_saopeng/, last accessed 7 March 2022.
23 See Collins (2000: 203).

References

Anderson, B. (1991). *Imagined Communities: Reflections on the Origin and Spread of Nationalism*. London: Verso.
Asad, T. (2013). "Free Speech, Blasphemy and Secular Critique." In T. Asad, W. Brown, J. Butler and S. Mahmood eds., *Is Critique Secular?* 14–57. New York: Fordham University Press.
Bankston, C. L. and Hidalgo, D. A. (2008). "Temple and Society in the New World: Theravada Buddhism and Social Order in North America." In P. Numrich ed., *North American Buddhists in Social Context*, 51–85. Leiden: Brill.
Bell, C. (1992). *Ritual Theory, Ritual Practice*. Oxford: Oxford University Press.
Bellah, R. N. (1991/1970). *Beyond Belief: Essays on Religion in a Post-traditionalist World*. Berkeley: University of California Press.
Bourdieu, P. (1977). *Outlines of a Theory of Practice*. Cambridge: Cambridge University Press.
Bourdieu, P. (1987). "Sociologues de la croyance et croyances de sociologues." *Archives de Sciences Sociales des Religions*, 32(63.1): 155–161.
Cadge, W. (2008). *Heartwood: The First Generation of Theravada Buddhism in America*. Chicago: University of Chicago Press.
Collins, S. (1997). *Nirvana and Other Buddhist Felicities*. Cambridge: Cambridge University Press.
Collins, S. (2000). "The Body in Theravada Buddhist Monasticism." In S. Coakley ed., *Religion and the Body*, 185–204. Cambridge: Cambridge University Press.
Crosby, K. (2014). *Theravada Buddhism: Continuity, Diversity, and Identity*. West Sussex: John Wiley and Sons, Inc.

Davis, E. W. (2016). "Binding Mighty Death: The Craft and Authority of the Rag Robe in Cambodian Ritual Technology." In *Deathpower: Buddhism's Ritual Imagination in Cambodia*, 138–158. New York: Columbia University Press.

De Voe, P. A. (2008). "The Role of Ethnic Leaders in the Refugee Community: A Case Study of the Lowland Lao in the American Midwest." In H. Ling ed., *Emerging Voices: Experiences of Underrepresented Asian Americans*, 52–69. New Brunswick: Rutgers University Press.

Do, A. (2021). "Elaborate Phone Tree Links Laotian Immigrants to COVID Info, One Another." *Los Angeles Times.* www.latimes.com/california/story/2021-05 -24/laotian-phone-tree-coronavirus, last accessed 3 March 2022.

Driscoll, C. (2022). "Live and Let Die: Spirits of White Christian Male Defiance in the Age of COVID-19." In S. Floyd-Thomas ed., *Religion, Race, and COVID-19: Confronting White Supremacy in the Pandemic*, 78–102. New York: New York University Press.

Foucault, M. (1988). "Technologies of the Self." In L. H. Martin ed., *Technologies of the Self: A Seminar with Michel Foucault*, 16–49. Amherst: University of Massachusetts Press.

Foucault, M. (1997). *Ethics: Subjectivity and Truth.* New York: The New Press.

Haselby, S. (2015). *The Origins of American Religious Nationalism.* Oxford: Oxford University Press.

Holt, J. C. (2017). *Theravada Traditions: Buddhist Ritual Cultures in Contemporary Southeast Asia and Sri Lanka.* Honolulu: University of Hawai'i Press.

Hong, M. K., Lau, C. Y. and Sharma, P. eds. (2021). *The Auntie Sewing Squad Guide to Mask Making, Radical Care, and Racial Justice.* Oakland: University of California Press.

Johnson, C. (2020). "While Some Try to Politicize Wearing Face Masks, For Me It's A Spiritual Practice." *Baptist News Global.* https://baptistnews.com/article/while -some-try-to-politicize-wearing-face-masks-for-me-its-a-spiritual-practice/, last accessed 31 January 2022.

Ladwig, P. (2017). "Contemporary Lao Buddhism. Ruptured Histories." In M. Jerryson ed., *The Oxford Encyclopedia of Contemporary Buddhism*, 274–296. New York: Oxford University Press.

Lee, J. H. X. (2015). *History of Asian Americans: Exploring Diverse Roots.* Santa Barbara: ABC-CLIO.

Lee, J. H. X. and the Center for Lao Studies. (2012). *Laotians in the San Francisco Bay Area.* Charleston: Arcadia Publishing.

Lupton, D., Southerton, C., Clark, M. and Watson, A. (2021). *The Face Mask in COVID Times.* Berlin and Boston: De Gruyter.

Mauss, M. (1966). *The Gift: Forms and Functions of Exchange in Archaic Societies.* Translated by Ian Cunnison. New York: Norton.

McLellan, J. and White, M. (2005). "Social Capital and Identity Politics among Asian Buddhists in Toronto." *Journal of International Migration & Integration*, 6(2): 235–253.

Merleau-Ponty, M. (1968). *The Visible and the Invisible.* Evanston: Northwestern University Press.

Mohan, U. (2016). "From Prayer Beads to the Mechanical Counter: The Negotiation of Chanting Practices within a Hindu Group." *Archives de Sciences Sociales des Religions*, 61(174): 191–212.

Mohan, U. (2019). *Clothing as Devotion in Contemporary Hinduism*. Leiden: Brill.

Mohan, U. (2021). "Devotion on the Home Altar as 'Efficacious Intimacy' in a Hindu Group." In U. Mohan and L. Douny eds., *The Material Subject: Rethinking Bodies and Objects in Motion*, 151–166. London and New York: Routledge.

Mohan, U. and Douny, L. eds. (2021). *The Material Subject: Rethinking Bodies and Objects in Motion*. London: Routledge.

Mohan, U. and Warnier, J.-P. (2017). "Marching the Devotional Subject: The Bodily-and-Material Cultures of Religion." *Journal of Material Culture*, 22(4): 369–384.

Monmouth University Polling Institute. (2020). *National: Protestors' Anger Justified Even If Actions May Not Be*. https://www.monmouth.edu/polling-institute/reports/monmouthpoll_us_060220/, last accessed 16 January 2022.

Morgan, D. (2007). "Seeing in Public: America as Imagined Community." In *The Lure of Images: A History of Religion and Visual Media in America*, 165–195; 282–296. London and New York: Routledge.

Morgan, D. (2015). *The Forge of Vision: A Visual History of Modern Christianity*. Berkeley: University of California Press.

Morgan, D. (2021). *The Thing About Religion: An Introduction to the Material Study of Religions*. Chapel Hill: UNC Press.

Ngaosyvathn, M. (1990). "Individual Soul, National Identity: The 'Baci-Sou Khuan' of the Lao." *Sojourn: Journal of Social Issues in Southeast Asia*, 5(2): 283–307.

Nyamnjoh, F. (2020). "Ubuntuism and Africa: Actualised, Misappropriated, Endangered, and Reappraised." *Alternation*, 36: 31–49.

Oliver, K. (2008). "Beyond Recognition: Merleau-Ponty and an Ethics of Vision." In G. Weiss ed., *Intertwinings: Interdisciplinary Encounters with Merleau-Ponty*, 131–151. Albany: State University of New York Press.

Oxford English Dictionary (2021). "Responsibility." In *Oxford English Dictionary*. Retrieved 22 February 2022, from www.oed.com/view/Entry/163862, last accessed 22 February 2022.

Parish, H. (2020). "The Absence of Presence and the Presence of Absence: Social Distancing, Sacraments, and the Virtual Religious Community during the COVID-19 Pandemic." *Religions*, 11(6): 276.

Promey, S. M., ed. (2014). *Sensational Religion: Sensory Cultures in Material Practice*. New Haven: Yale University Press.

Reed, E. D. (2021). "Responsibility." In T. Winright ed., *T&T Clark Handbook of Christian Ethics*, 111–120. London: T&T Clark.

Rey, T. (2007). *Bourdieu on Religion: Imposing Faith and Legitimacy*. New York: Routledge.

Riggs, D. E. (2017). "Golden Robe or Rubbish Robe? Interpretations of the Transmitted Robe in Tokugawa Period Zen Buddhist Thought." In P. D. Winfield and S. Heine ed., *Zen and Material Culture*, 197–228. New York: Oxford University Press.

Stoddart, E. (2021). "Retreat, Rebuke, Recite: Outliers in Church Responses to the Current COVID-19 Pandemic." *Practical Theology*, 14(1–2): 8–21.

Strenski, I. (2020). "Why Durkheim Really Thought That Buddhism Was a 'Religion'." *Religion*, 50(4): 653–670.

Tambiah, S. J. (2013). *Culture, Thought, and Social Action: An Anthropological Perspective.* Cambridge and London: Harvard University Press.

Tanabe, W. J. (2003). "Robes and Clothing." In R. E. Buswell, Jr. ed., *Encyclopedia of Buddhism, Vol. 2*, 731–735. New York: Macmillan Reference.

Vajirananavarorasa, S. P. M. S. C. K. P. (1973). *The Entrance to the Vinaya, Vol. 2.* Bangkok: Mahamakut Rajavidyalaya Press.

Van Esterik, P. (1992). *Taking Refuge: Lao Buddhists in North America.* Tempe: Arizona State University.

Van Esterik, P. (1999). "Ritual and the Performance of Buddhist Identity Among Lao Buddhists in North America." In C. Queen and D. R. Williams ed., *American Buddhism: Methods and Findings in Recent Scholarship*, 57–68. London and New York: Taylor and Francis.

Wallace, J. (2020). "Masking: Response-ability, in Unsteady, Broken Breaths." *Philosophy & Rhetoric*, 53(3): 336–343.

Warnier, J.-P. (2006). "Inside and Outside: Surfaces and Containers." In C. Tilley, W. Keane, S. Küchler, M. Rowlands and P. Spyer eds., *Handbook of Material Culture*, 186–195. London: Sage.

Weber, M. (2001). *The Protestant Ethic and the Spirit of Capitalism.* New York: Routledge.

Whitehead, A. L. and Perry, S. L. (2020). *Taking America Back for God: Christian Nationalism in the United States.* New York: Oxford University Press.

Wilson, S. M. and Peterson, L. C. (2002). "The Anthropology of Online Communities." *Annual Review of Anthropology*, 31(1): 449–467.

Winter, J. (2021). "The Promise of Immanent Critique." In W. F. Sullivan and E. S. Hurd eds., *Theologies of American Exceptionalism.* Bloomington: Indiana University Press, https://publish.iupress.indiana.edu/projects/TAE2019_theologies, last accessed 11 March 2022.

5 Conclusion

Imaginaries of masking and unmasking

Introduction

A photo of a New York city pavement taken a few months after the first novel coronavirus outbreak in 2020 captures a series of turning points through the impact of hundreds of feet (Figure 5.1). The image shows a trail of earth amongst the grass and weeds, marking peoples' new pursuits as well as displacement from previous spaces and routines. Even during this time of immense uncertainty, the path shows the desire of people to maintain pre-existing habits. It veers around trees and uneven terrain, marking the landscape with the prevailing wisdom at that time—the requisite six feet of social distancing between people. The photo itself does not feature many people as it was taken when a few gyms and workplaces had reopened, and people could find other venues for exercise. However, the road is remarkably empty of vehicles, a pattern that would continue for many more months, marking the apocalyptic silence that people had come to associate with the pandemic. Even as people adopted the language of "shelter-in-place" and "lockdown," reflecting prison and war protocols, it would take a while for them to realize the full extent to which their lives had been transformed.

The practices explored in this book were part of an attempt to understand how the pandemic became a social space of action and engagement. In this world, subjects and objects were co-produced via the "efficacious intimacy" (Mohan 2019, 2021) of bodies and materials, and compelling notions of community, labor, and care were made real. Designers, artists, educators, and members of faith and civic engagement communities both shaped their environment and were shaped by "techniques of the self" and biopolitical power. They were quintessential material subjects since they designed and sewed while coping with limitations of objects and techniques. Simultaneously, they, like other Americans, were subject to wider public hygiene practices and mandates, and debates about autonomy and

DOI: 10.4324/9781003244103-6

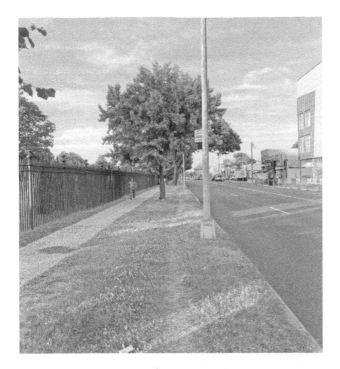

Figure 5.1 A path created by runners over the first few months of pandemic lockdown. Brooklyn, New York. June 2020. Photo by author.

bodily freedom. The images that makers encountered around their work were folded into their worldmaking as they relied on beliefs, affects, and emotions to navigate gaps, contestations, and tensions. It was within this paradigm that mask making and usage were studied as activities of worldmaking.

The virus and practices of its containment were approached as part of a "governmentality of containers" (Warnier 2007: 131)[1] through actions of opening and closing, attaching and detaching, and incorporating and dis-incorporating. Such practices of the state in its various forms kept certain people and entities in while excluding or keeping others out, for instance, through monitoring of national boundaries, citizens' physical bodies, and supporting certain non-governmental and community groups over others. Even as pandemic protocols and support systems were created with a normative American in mind, citizens' claims to equity in the eyes of the state were belied by the growing realization that "privileges of subjectivation" (Bertrand 2021) allowed a segment of the population to survive and even thrive during the pandemic. Ordering and disciplining was thus a variable phenomenon influenced by class, race, and occupation, and an exploration of peoples' belief-making processes indicated that its effects extended to what Americans chose to contain or connect with as values in their daily lives. As diverse "material subjects" (Mohan and Douny eds. 2021) engaged in living, peoples' power to move through physical and social spaces manifested as varied abilities to grasp and navigate scapes, and respond to the possibilities afforded by the milieu.

Dynamics of masking and unmasking

Concepts of containment, connection, and territorialization were used in this book as a means of analyzing pandemic responses and effects via value-laden exchanges. These ideas were drawn from Appadurai's (1996) study of globalization and Warnier's (2007) exploration of bodily techniques in the Cameroonian kingdom of Mankon. In exploring unmasking, their study of how communities form can be juxtaposed with Harvey's[2] (2005: 65) articulation of how late capitalism relies on a continual process of "enclosure," replacing mutual responsibility with individual ownership and segregation. By contrast, collective action in the form of food banks, Black Lives Matter protests, public art projects, and mask sewing demonstrates a "politics of commoning" (Kirwan et al. 2015: 2–3) or how ways of living together could resist the privatization and individualization of life. It is from this relational angle, and by connecting uncertainty to care, that the autonomous American self is challenged.

Beliefs in U.S. exceptionalism were shaken by the COVID-19 pandemic, revealing the fragile state of the framework that seemingly cohered the nation. After experiencing infectious variants of SARS-CoV-2, such as Delta (mid-late 2021) and Omicron (2021-2022), it was hoped that Americans would finally regain the freedom to live without mandates on masking, entering public spaces as they wished, and not having to show digital "vaccine passports" or other forms of identifications when they traveled within or between states. That is, Americans would regain the freedom to move when and how they liked even as the rest of the world contended with ongoing waves of the virus and vaccine inequity. On the occasion of his first State of the Union address[3] and during the month of the pandemic's second anniversary, President Joe Biden stated that COVID-19 no longer controlled the lives of American people. He also stated that the virus could mutate and spread, and so "we have to stay on guard." This aspect of staying vigilant competed with the push for normalcy[4] as people celebrated the possibility of going "mask free" and being able to enter public spaces without restrictions.

Folds of pandemic subjectivation

Responsivity has been explored as a process of worldmaking that constantly folds (Deleuze 1988: 94) in affects and subjectivities through a meeting of the external and internal. A graphic illustration of pivoting as a means of folding in prior worlds was the way costumers worked to make and distribute masks. During a time of changing scientific conclusions and misinformation, mask stitchers used existing tools, gestures, and cognitive approaches to make do, manifesting their response-ability. In doing so, they connected—even if temporarily—the flux of disparate imaginaries. With the mask's plenum acting as a liminal space of exchange via inhalation and exhalation, breathing came to symbolize not just a fraught activity but responsivity to the virus' effects, including the potential transgression of individual and social boundaries.

In New York city, where I observed the pandemic's (un)folding, some fled the city either temporarily or permanently, while frontline and health care workers faced the virus' ravaging effects in hospitals, nursing homes, and assisted living facilities. Class and occupation played a significant role in who was exposed to the virus and who could pivot to working from home. Those who had to show up for work in person and those who held multiple jobs rolled the dice of being infected more frequently, thereby bringing the virus home to their unvaccinated families. Like Americans elsewhere, the city's inhabitants worried about elderly parents, the rising toll of sickness and deaths in the extended family, including those in other countries, and how children would continue their schooling. What people valued and how they realized this in pandemic responses became part of the shifting culture around a mutating virus. Deaths from the virus have been normalized, contact tracing and quarantine policies are discouraged, and there is skepticism about further COVID-19 funding from the government. If there was a period of pause caused by the virus entering the U.S., there is now a "Sisyphean cycle of panic and neglect"[5] raising questions about preparedness for the next pandemic.

In successive waves of the virus and its variants, New York city went through soft lockdowns, and at the time of writing unmasking is taking place at an accelerated pace. A follow-up with Maria, the young Mexican-American woman first met in Chapter 1, provides a brief idea of the issues at play. In December 2021, despite double masking, Maria caught the highly contagious Omicron variant during a Christmas party with extended family. She was distraught about the possibility that she could have transmitted the virus to restaurant staff but, fortunately, that did not happen. One might say that her concern for the workers was self-interest motivated by the desire to keep the business running, but it is precisely this kind of relationality that was surprisingly missing in many instances. The phenomenon of diminishing or dismissing the pandemic effects so as to marginalize the importance of care for both oneself and others relates to powerful imaginaries including Americans' view of the government and health care system, active disinformation, as well as a belief in certain peoples' absolute control over their bodies. The U.S.' segregationist history and zero-sum paradigm (McGhee 2021) also lend themselves to ways of thinking that allocate blame for the spread of disease to specific racial groups, thus moving the responsibility for care solely onto a normative individual or group. In public spaces, the conflicts that result from these approaches are what the Centers for Disease Control and Prevention (CDC) terms broadly as occupational or workplace hazards.[6]

On the day I conversed with Maria, her mother Rosa had been stressed by interactions with customers and pre-existing health problems, and had been encouraged to take a day off from work to rest and take care of herself. Maria's younger siblings who were still in school preferred to take virtual classes to stay safe since new rules did not require students to quarantine even if directly exposed to those with COVID-19. Her godmother who worked at a daycare center was finding the de-mandating process difficult, worried about the hardship for vulnerable children under the age of five who could not be vaccinated as well as their parents who could not afford to fall sick by contracting the virus from their children and missing work. In the meantime, customers continued to arrive at the family's restaurant expecting to be accommodated without masks, and Maria and Rosa could only request that they mask to protect the workers.

Part of the critique of care in the U.S. is how propositions of caring for and caring about, including the future, are ultimately essentialized as individualized care for one's self or family. Even as the state makes appeals to ideals of community, the vision of American freedom that is valorized is one that relies on individual responsibility and autonomy. However, care is realized in social contexts such as schools and businesses, as seen in the case of Maria's restaurant, making it a source of conflict when the people involved do not see the same practice as care but as a burden. Further, what such conflicts reveal is that the notion of the "social" itself has to be constantly re-evaluated for what or who is excluded and included. At the time of writing, the subway was one of the few public places in New York city where masking was still mandated (Figure 5.2). The cheery, yellow sign with cartoon characters gesturing a "thumbs up" urged commuters to take care of each other reciprocally and stop the spread of the virus. The figure on the left side is double-masked, a recommended practice during the Delta variant surge in 2021.

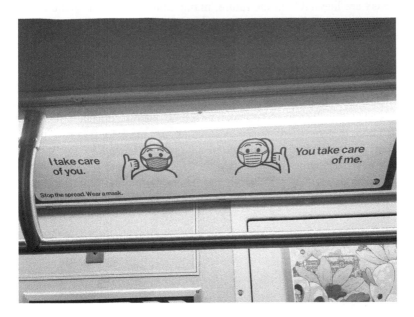

Figure 5.2 A masking sign inside a subway train. New York city. September 2021.
    Photo by author.

The pandemic–endemic–syndemic scape

The logic of recovery that is contained in terms such as "new normal"
and "next normal"[7] assumes a significant break between a pre- and post-
pandemic U.S. while telling us little about the "countless ways for a disease to go endemic."[8] Despite calls for imaginative ways of thinking about
unmasking, the future seems to be business as usual via a prioritizing of
the (management of the) economy *as* normalcy. Simultaneously, a roadmap authored by scholars and experts, including six of President Biden's
16-member COVID-19 Advisory Board, noted that the pandemic has "dis-
proportionately impacted people of color, rural communities, tribal lands,
and other underserved groups and locations, exacerbating existing health
disparities" (Albarracín et al. 2022: 19). Even while factoring in viral unpre-
dictability and "the impossibility of securing the body politic" (Keck et al.
eds. 2019: 1) in a globalized world, it is unclear how such socio-economic
inequities are to be avoided in the future; what we need is a mixture of long-
term structural solutions as well as being attentive to, and supporting, people's emergent thinking and practices.[9] If SARS and other respiratory viral

outbreaks are inevitable in the future, maintaining reciprocal relationships of care at the everyday level and simply knowing *how* to move or adapt pre-existing ways to respond will be essential.

The "prism of incompleteness" (Nyamnjoh 2022, Introduction)[10] is a productive way to think about the generativity of pandemic flux, and the ways some makers used their agency and skills to foreground the importance of the social, providing compelling alternatives to the autonomous American. For instance, this display of masks on a clothes line on a pavement is based on the honor system where passersby can pick up a mask for free and "pay it forward" by donating to a local mutual-aid group (Figure 5.3). By framing making and distributing practices via the lens of care and responsibility, I do not mean to say that worldmaking is inherently a good or uniform process, but that material, practical, and affective engagement is necessary for

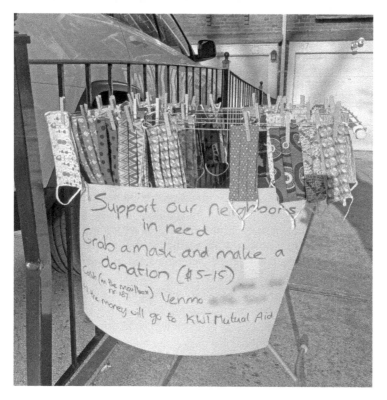

Figure 5.3 A mutual-aid sign offering masks. Brooklyn, New York. April 2021. Photo by author.

beliefs to emerge as compelling forces of reals. In actuality, the experiences and perceptions of several makers showed that even within communities of care, people took to sewing in different ways, motivated by different agendas and the needs of diverse recipients. The designers, stitchers, and faith and community leaders highlighted in this book were certainly aware of how their work, directly or indirectly, changed the world. Some were also engaged with challenging narratives of whose bodies were most deserving of protection. They refined value systems (un)consciously and prioritized a relational model of society that could be sustained despite physical distancing—testing and adapting earlier ways of doing things to deal with the novel coronavirus. (Indeed, the pandemic subjects encountered in this book are also digital subjects, a topic that deserves its own in-depth study.) If the flexibility of ideas and practices that emerged during this time are not to be simply re-absorbed into routines,[11] it is important to recognize both the political and socio-economic forces that exist as well as how worlds are imagined and made real, including the types of conflicts and contestations.

While hoping for permanent, low level rates of the virus in the future, a counterfactual history helps imagine[12] how things may have been different at key early turning points and shows, via a plausible alternative path, what future goals might be. These include accepting from the start that transmission could take place without symptoms, recognizing airborne spread, the importance of clusters, and the need to increase vaccine supply and distribute it equitably. A vision of the "next normal," health professionals advise, must be accompanied by new protocols including isolated periods of masking in outbreaks areas and seasonal vaccination against new variants. It is hoped that the pandemic will become endemic eventually but with approximately 1 million deaths and a total of approximately 80 million cases in the U.S. by late March 2022,[13] it is the syndemic aspects—social, economic, and health inequalities—that seem most difficult to acknowledge or resolve. While new variants are watched closely and defense systems, such as N95 masks, vaccines, and medicines, are built up for future SARS-CoV-2 pandemics, the type of affective, political, and spiritual work needed to care for people is daunting. Such labor only seems sustainable in a society that acknowledges the incompleteness of its subjects. A place where humans are social beings, constantly engaged in relationships of "debt and indebtedness" (Nymanjoh 2022, Chapter 3, Section 2, para. 3) with each other, transcendental forces, and viruses.

Uncertainty, in and of itself, is not necessarily a bad or negative state. Pandemic pause exercised "revelatory power" as interruption (Dawney 2013: 641) and, as this book explored, practices both contained and connected Americans as diverse subjects. The imaginary of "pause and pivot" engaged differing folds of responsivity and responsibility. This was not simply a question of being for or against masks and vaccines, and indicated the complexity of how power flowed through intersecting scapes of media, public policy, health care, politics, and religion. Simultaneously, the pandemic unsettled previously cherished images and provided people opportunities to reconsider and identify what mattered to them. Makers not only sewed cloth masks but helped lay paths of response-ability to the future by identifying and realizing care as image, object, and action.

Notes

1 Warnier describes this as a Foucauldian "techniques of self" applied to human and social bodies.
2 See Harvey (2005 in Kirwan et al. 2015: 2) for how capital expands to replace social relations of mutual responsibility.
3 https://www.nytimes.com/2022/03/01/us/politics/biden-sotu-transcript.html, last accessed 14 March 2022. He also emphasized using vaccinations and, if needed, antiviral treatments.
4 See letter by heads of American airlines at https://www.reuters.com/world/us /us-airline-ceos-urge-biden-lift-covid-mask-mandate-letter-2022-03-23, last accessed 25 March 2022; and speech by Mayor Eric Adams, https://www .nytimes.com/2022/03/07/nyregion/nyc-school-mask-mandate.html, last accessed 14 March 2022.
5 See Yong (2022), https://www.theatlantic.com/health/archive/2022/03/congress -covid-spending-bill/627090, last accessed 31 March 2022.
6 See strategies to deal with vaccination avoidance and anti-masking violence in retail spaces. https://www.cdc.gov/coronavirus/2019-ncov/community/work-places-businesses/, last accessed on 29 March 2022.
7 https://www.covidroadmap.org, last accessed 15 March 2022,
8 See Stern and Wu (2022), https://www.theatlantic.com/health/archive/2022/02/ endemicity-means-nothing/621423, last accessed 31 March 22.
9 Although it is beyond the scope of this chapter to do this, such assumptions must be critiqued with every new event—viral or human—as they indicate how practices shape worlds through the imaginary of unmasking.
10 The late Nigerian writer Amos Tutuola's depictions of incompleteness (Nyamnjoh 2015) are connected to the populism of former President Donald Trump (Nyamnjoh 2022) and the African concept of *Ubuntu* (Nyamnjoh 2015) as a social organizing principle, where relationships are constantly in motion and things move to maintain a balance of reciprocity between oneself and others.
11 See Berlant (2011: 196).
12 See Tufekci (2022).
13 https://covid.cdc.gov/covid-data-tracker/, last accessed 14 March 2022.

References

Albarracín, D., Bedford, T., Bollyky, T., Borio, L., Bright, R., Brosseau, L. M., … Wherry, E. J. (2022). *Getting to and Sustaining the Next Normal: A Roadmap for Living with COVID*. www.covidroadmap.org, last accessed 29 March 2022.

Appadurai, A. (1996). *Modernity at Large: Cultural Dimensions of Globalization.* Minnesota: University of Minnesota Press.

Berlant, L. (2011). *Cruel Optimism.* Durham: Duke University Press.

Bertrand, R. (2021). "Chronicles of a Moral War: Ascetic Subjectivation and Formation of the Javanese State." In U. Mohan and L. Douny eds., *The Material Subject: Rethinking Bodies and Objects in Motion,* 121–134. London: Routledge.

Dawney, L. (2013). "The Interruption: Investigating Subjectivation and Affect." *Environment and Planning D: Society and Space,* 31(4): 628–644.

Deleuze, G. (1988). *Foucault.* Minneapolis: University of Minnesota Press.

Harvey, D. (2005). *A Brief History of Neoliberalism.* Oxford: Oxford University Press.

Keck, F., Kelly, A. H. and Lynteris, C. eds. (2019). *The Anthropology of Epidemics.* London and New York: Routledge.

Kirwan, S., Dawney, L. and Brigstocke, J. eds. (2015). *Space, Power and the Commons: The Struggle for Alternative Futures.* New York: Routledge.

McGhee, H. (2021). *The Sum of Us: What Racism Costs Everyone and How We Can Prosper Together.* New York: Random House.

Mohan, U. (2019). *Clothing as Devotion in Contemporary Hinduism.* Leiden: Brill.

Mohan, U. (2021). "Devotion on the Home Altar as 'Efficacious Intimacy' in a Hindu Group." In U. Mohan and L. Douny eds. *The Material Subject: Rethinking Bodies and Objects in Motion,* 151–166. London and New York: Routledge.

Mohan, U. and Douny, L. eds. (2021). *The Material Subject: Rethinking Bodies and Objects in Motion.* London: Routledge.

Nyamnjoh, F. (2015). "Amos Tutuola and the Elusiveness of Completeness." *Wiener Zeitschrift für kritische Afrikastudien (Vienna Journal of African Studies),* 29(15): 1–47.

Nyamnjoh, F. (2022). *Incompleteness: Donald Trump, Populism and Citizenship.* Bamenda: Langaa RPCIG. Kindle Edition.

Stern, J. and Wu, K. J. (2022). "Endemicity is Meaningless." *The Atlantic.* https://www.theatlantic.com/health/archive/2022/02/endemicity-means-nothing/621423/, last accessed 31 March 2022.

Tufekci, Z. (2022). "How Millions of Lives Might Have Been Saved from Covid-19." *The New York Times.* https://www.nytimes.com/2022/03/11/opinion/covid-health-pandemic.html, last accessed 15 March 2022.

Warnier, J.-P. (2007). *The Pot-King: The Body and Technologies of Power.* Leiden: Brill.

Yong, Ed. (2022). "America is Zooming Through the Pandemic Panic-Neglect Cycle." https://www.theatlantic.com/health/archive/2022/03/congress-covid-spending-bill/627090, last accessed 31 March 2022.

Index

124   *Index*

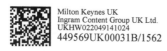
Milton Keynes UK
Ingram Content Group UK Ltd.
UKHW022049141024
449569UK00031B/1562